Coloring Guide to Human Anatomy

THIRD EDITION

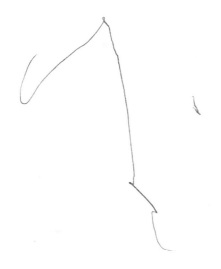

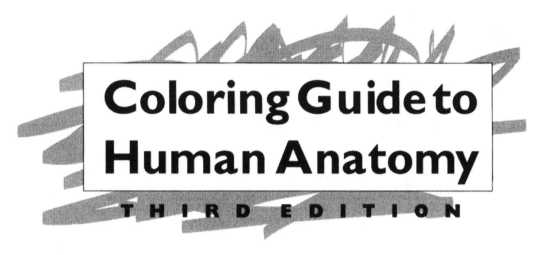

Coloring Guide to Human Anatomy
THIRD EDITION

T. Alan Twietmeyer, PhD

Professor
Department of Kinesiology
Concordia College
Ann Arbor, MI

Thomas McCracken, MS

Vice President, Product and Development
Visible Productions
Fort Collins, CO

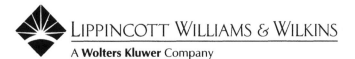

LIPPINCOTT WILLIAMS & WILKINS
A **Wolters Kluwer** Company

Philadelphia · Baltimore · New York · London
Buenos Aires · Hong Kong · Sydney · Tokyo

Editor: Robert Anthony
Managing Editor: Ulita Lushnycky
Marketing Manager: Aimee Sirmon
Production Manager: Susan Rockwell

Copyright © 2001 Lippincott Williams & Wilkins

351 West Camden Street
Baltimore, Maryland 21201-2436 USA

530 Walnut Street
Philadelphia, Pennsylvania 19106 USA

The publisher is not responsible (as a matter of product liability, negligence, or otherwise) for any injury resulting from any material contained herein. This publication contains information relating to general principles of medical care, which should not be construed as specific instructions for individual patients. Manufacturers' product information and package inserts should be reviewed for current information, including contraindications, dosages, and precautions.

Printed in the United States of America.

Library of Congress Cataloging-in-Publication Data

Twietmeyer, Alan.
    Coloring guide to human anatomy / T. Alan Twietmeyer, Thomas McCracken.—3rd ed.
        p. cm.
    Includes index.
    ISBN 13: 978-0-7817-3042-6
    ISBN 10: 0-7817-3042-2
        1. Human anatomy—Atlases. 2. Coloring books. I. McCracken, Thomas II. Title.

QM25 .T85 2001
611—dc21   2001029396

The publishers have made every effort to trace the copyright holders for borrowed material. If they have inadvertently overlooked any, they will be pleased to make the necessary arrangements at the first opportunity.

To purchase additional copies of this book call our customer service department at **(800) 638-3030** or fax orders to **(301) 824-7390**. International customers should call **(301) 714-2324**.

14 15 16 17 18 19 20

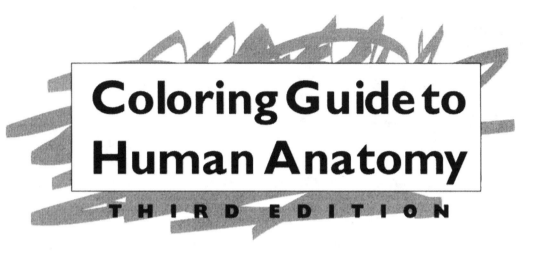

Coloring Guide to Human Anatomy

THIRD EDITION

T. Alan Twietmeyer, PhD

Professor
Department of Kinesiology
Concordia College
Ann Arbor, MI

Thomas McCracken, MS

Vice President, Product and Development
Visible Productions
Fort Collins, CO

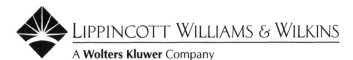

LIPPINCOTT WILLIAMS & WILKINS
A **Wolters Kluwer** Company
Philadelphia · Baltimore · New York · London
Buenos Aires · Hong Kong · Sydney · Tokyo

Editor: Robert Anthony
Managing Editor: Ulita Lushnycky
Marketing Manager: Aimee Sirmon
Production Manager: Susan Rockwell

351 West Camden Street
Baltimore, Maryland 21201-2436 USA

530 Walnut Street
Philadelphia, Pennsylvania 19106 USA

Printed in the United States of America.

Library of Congress Cataloging-in-Publication Data

Twietmeyer, Alan.
  Coloring guide to human anatomy / T. Alan Twietmeyer, Thomas McCracken.—3rd ed.
    p. cm.
  Includes index.
  ISBN 13: 978-0-7817-3042-6
  ISBN 10: 0-7817-3042-2
    1. Human anatomy—Atlases. 2. Coloring books. I. McCracken, Thomas II. Title.

QM25 .T85 2001
611—dc21   2001029396

To purchase additional copies of this book call our customer service department at **(800) 638-3030** or fax orders to **(301) 824-7390**. International customers should call **(301) 714-2324**.

14 15 16 17 18 19 20

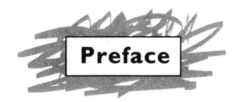

Preface

GOAL

The goal of this new edition is to provide learners with an enjoyable, enlightening, and invigorating format for the study of human gross anatomy. Toward this goal this edition embraces substantial changes. The approach of the text has been changed to a systemic model, many more interactive opportunities for writing and coloring have been added; illustrations have been added, deleted, or modified; and auxiliary panels accompany many of the included illustrations. Textual and layout changes have been made as well. Throughout this text instructional material will be presented on the left panel and illustrative material on the right, allowing for greater ease and clarity of reading, notation, and coloring. We remain focused toward the goal of making the learning of human gross anatomy more meaningful. Anatomy is a study of self and should be fun! We have enjoyed creating this text and hope every reader will enjoy using it!

AUDIENCE

This text is not self-limiting to courses taught with or without laboratories or to certain groups of students. The most obvious audience includes students in allied health fields: kinesiology, athletic training, occupational and physical therapy; and majors in biology, zoology, or art. However, enough factual information is presented in a concise and clear manner to make this an appropriate review source for learners in medicine, dentistry, or nursing.

APPROACH AND RATIONALE

The most important approach of this text is that of active learning. The format is didactic, as if in person with the learner. Throughout the text the learner is guided to fill in a blank, color a structure, or color an identity bar next to a structure, all providing a psychomotor component to learning. Opportunities are provided for listing attachments and innervation of muscles, movements allowed at various joints, and labeling. Throughout the text are sections entitled **FOR REVIEW AND THOUGHT, JUST FOR FUN,** and **ACTIVE LEARNING** in which the learner is to actively review key items individually or with a partner. The overall intent is to involve the learner thoroughly in the material.

In ordering the material we take a 'regional approach to systems'. For example, study of the skeletal system will be conducted regionally: appendicular skeleton (upper limb, lower limb, and associated girdles), vertebral column, ribs, and face and skull.

The left panel text/right panel illustration format of this guide is entirely new and is a key to achieving its goal. This approach puts words and pictures together, promoting earlier concept formation and subsequent understanding. The learner has nearly immediate access to facts without searching through voluminous textual material. It is our hope that this approach will provide teacher and student with an enjoyable and challenging foray into the study of gross human anatomy.

The ideas and methods incorporated in this edition have incubated in our minds for many years, kept warm by frequent discussion and criticism and the advice of colleagues and readers. The ideas for additions, deletions, and improvements came from all of these sources. We thank everyone. We would especially like to thank Gale Mueller for providing beautiful illustrations for this edition.

T. Alan Twietmeyer
Ann Arbor, Michigan

Thomas McCracken
Ft. Collins, Colorado

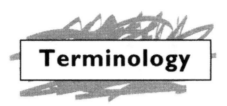

Terminology

TO THE LEARNER

The teaching and learning of anatomy are communicated through a language derived from a variety of sources, though mainly from Greek and Latin. This page provides you with a listing of common root words, prefixes, and suffixes which you will encounter in your studies. Each listing gives the Latin (L) or Greek (G) derivation and a sample usage. This list is by no means complete, so be prepared to add to it. Use the language of anatomy to aid your learning. Practice "Anglicizing" the Latin or Greek terms, for example: triceps brachii = three-headed muscle of the arm. Your success in learning anatomy will be closely linked to your success in using the language.

Source	Example	Term
a-(an-)	G. without, not	anemia
ab-	L. from	abduct
acro	G. extremity, tip	acromion process
ad-	L. to, toward	adduct
aden-	G. gland	adenoid
adipo-	L. fat	adipose
ambi-	L. both	ambidextrous
ante-	L. before, forward	anteversion
anti-	G. against	antiseptic
arth-(arthro-)	G. a joint	arthritis
auto-	G. self	autonomic
bi	L. two, double	bilateral
-blast	G. germ, bud	fibroblast
brachi-(brachion)-	G. arm	brachial artery
brachium	L. arm	
brevis	L. short	peroneus brevis
capit (caput)	L. head	semispinalis capitis
cervix	L. neck	cervix of uterus
chondro-	L. cartilage	chondrocyte
circum-	L. around, about	circumflex
-clast	G. to break	osteoclast
contra-	L. against, opposed	contralateral
costa	L. rib	intercostal
crus	L. leg	talocrural joint
crux	L. cross	cruciate ligament
delta	G. triangle	deltoid
derm	g. skin	dermatome
di-	G. through, completely	diagnosis
dis-	L. separation	dissect
ect-	G. outside	ectoderm
-ectomy	G. excision, removal	hysterectomy
end-(ent-)	G. within	endothelium

Source	Example	Term
epi-	G. upon	epicondyle
ex-(exo-)	G. & L. out	exocrine
extra-	L. beyond, outward	extracellular
gastr-(gastro-)	G. tissue	gastritis
hist-(histo-)	G. tissue	histology
hyal-(hyalo-)	G. glossy, clear	hyaline cartilage
hydro-	G. water	hydrocephalus
hyper-	G. above, over	hypertrophy
hypo-	G. under, less	hypothalamus
im-,in-	L. into	incision
im-,in-	G. negation, not	immature, involuntary
infra-	L. below	infraspinatus
inter-	L. between	intercondylar
intr-(intra-)	L. within	intravenous
ipsi	L. self; same	ipsilateral
linea	L. line	linea alba
macro-	G. large	macrophage
medi-	G. middle	median
meta-	G. changed, beyond	metatarsal
micro-	G. small	microbiology
myo-	G. muscle	myology
nephr-	G. kidney	nephron
-oid	G. line, appearance, form	adenoid
para-	G. beside	paravertebral
peri-	G. around	perichondrium
-physis	G. to grow	physical
post-	L. after, behind	postnatal
pre-	L. before, in front of	preganglionic
pro-	G. before, in front of	prosencephalon
ram-	L. branch	ramus
re-	L. again, back	recurrent
rect-	L. straight	rectus femoris
ren-	L. kidney	renal
retro-	L. back, backward	retroverted
-sect	L. to cut	dissect
sub-	L. under	subdural
super-	L. over, excessive	superficial
supra-	L. above	supraorbital
sym,syn-	G. together	symphysis, synthesis
teres	L. round	ligamentum teres
trans-	L. across, through, beyond	transfusion
tub(er)	L. swelling; node	tubercle
tome	G. cut	appendectomy
ultra-	L. beyond, excess	ultrastructure
vas	L. duct, vessel	vas deferens
vent-(ventr-)	L. belly	ventral

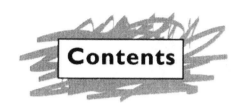

Contents

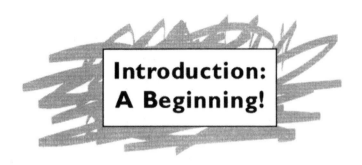

Introduction: A Beginning!

Your study of human anatomy must begin with an understanding of descriptive terminology; one which will carry through your learning and provide 'geographic' clues to movements, functions, and positions of various structures. If you were taking a journey in a foreign country you would prepare by learning some elements of that country's language, as well as descriptive terms to aid in your travel. The same is true for your journey through the human body! A list of terminology is found previous to this introduction (page viii). Use this list to begin your familiarization with the language of anatomy.

An important concept upon which terminology is based is that of the 'anatomical position' (FIGURE Intro.1). From this position the body, and its movements, can be described using a series of paired terms with planes and axes as guides. These paired terms are:

anterior/posterior – front/back
  ex. the tip of the nose is anterior to the forehead; the forehead is posterior to the tip of the nose
note: the terms ventral and dorsal are also used to describe anterior/posterior
  ex. ventral and dorsal interossei muscles
superior/inferior – closer to/further from the head
  ex. the shoulder is superior to the elbow; the elbow is inferior to the shoulder
medial/lateral – closer to/further from the middle of a structure
  ex. the eye is medial to the ear; the ear is lateral to the eye
proximal/distal – closer to/further from the beginning of a structure
  ex. the shoulder is proximal to the elbow; the elbow is distal to the shoulder
superficial/deep – closer to/further from the surface
  ex. the sternum is superficial to the heart; the heart is deep to the sternum
ipsilateral/contralateral – same side/opposite side
  ex. the right knee and right elbow are ipsilateral; the right knee and left elbow are contralateral

PLANES

A sagittal plane is one that divides the body into right and left portions. If this division occurs in the exact middle of the body it is called a midsagittal, or median plane. On FIGURE Intro.1a outline the midsagittal plane in red.

A frontal plane is one that divides the body into anterior and posterior portions. On FIGURE Intro.1b outline the frontal plane in yellow.

A transverse plane divides the body into superior and inferior portions. Outline the transverse plane in FIGURE Intro.1c in blue.

AXES

Movement of the body occurs about axes of rotation through the planes already described. Flexion and extension are opposite movements and occur in a sagittal plane about a transverse axis. Flexion is movement anteriorly and extension is movement posteriorly. On FIGURE Intro.1a color the arrows purple to indicate flexion and extension.

Abduction and adduction are also opposite movements but they occur in a frontal plane about a sagittal axis. Abduction is movement away and adduction is movement toward. In FIGURE Intro.1b color the arrows orange to indicate abduction and adduction.

Rotation occurs in a transverse plane about a frontal axis. No opposite descriptor exists for rotation of the head, but in the limbs medial and lateral rotation are described. In FIGURE Intro.1c color the arrows green.

Red + blue = purple (flexion/extension)

Red + yellow = orange (abduction/adduction)

Yellow + blue = green (rotation)

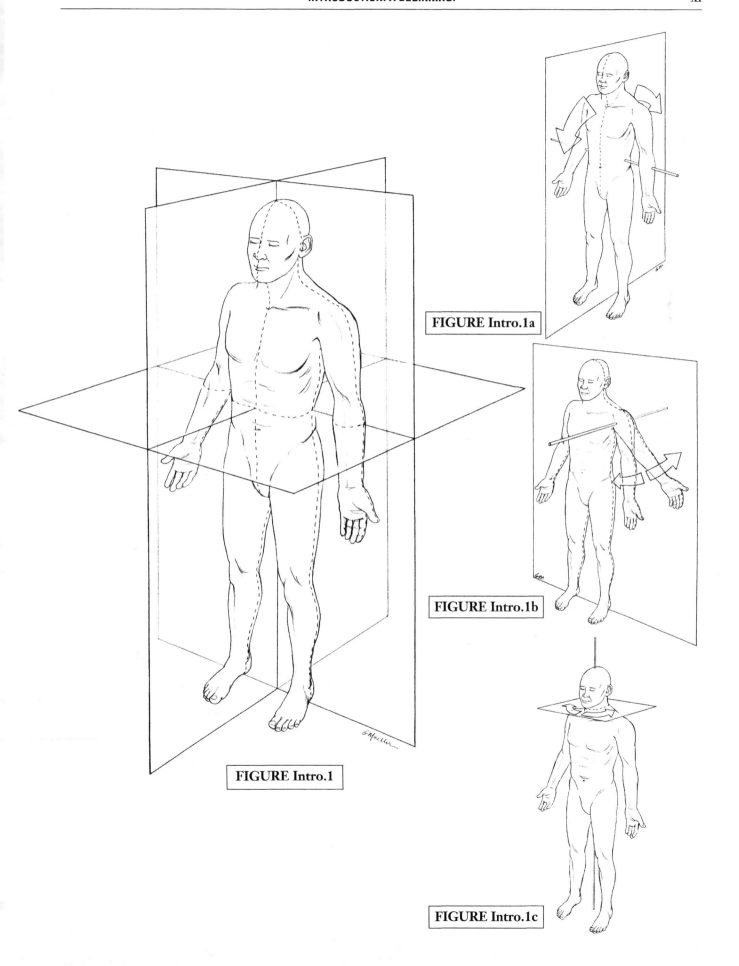

FIGURE Intro.1a

FIGURE Intro.1b

FIGURE Intro.1

FIGURE Intro.1c

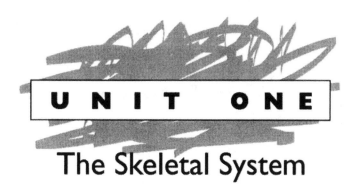

UNIT ONE

The Skeletal System

The adult human skeleton is composed of 206 individual bones which, for classification purposes, may be grouped into axial and appendicular portions. The axial (axis, central, core) skeleton includes the skull, vertebral column, sternum, and ribs. Trace the outline of the axial skeleton in black. The appendicular (attached, added, appended) skeleton includes the bones of the limbs and their appropriate girdles. Trace the outline of the appendicular skeleton in red-orange. The pectoral and pelvic girdles serve to join the upper and lower limbs, respectively, to the axial skeleton.

The skeleton is involved in five major bodily functions: hemopoiesis, mineral reservoir, support, protection, and movement. Not all bones have these functions equally. This fact, and their location in the body, determine their shape. A simple classification scheme for bones is as follows:

Long – have a body (shaft) and two somewhat expanded ends; found in the limbs
Short – have no long axis; found in ankle and wrist
Flat – ribs; sternum; bones of cranium
Irregular – vertebrae; scapulae; pelvis; facial

On FIGURES Ia Anterior, Ib Posterior, and Ic Lateral color the bones in this manner:

Long bones – brown
Short bones – light brown
Flat bones – sky blue
Irregular – yellow-green

As you study bones get into the habit of mentally classifying them by shape, location, and function. Bones possess certain landmarks caused by muscle attachments, passage of blood vessels or nerves, association with tendons, and union with other bones. The following terms describe landmarks on bones. As you encounter these terms write in the definition and an example of a bone possessing such a landmark.

Term	Definition	Example
spine	an abrupt/pointed projection	scapula
process		
tubercle		
tuberosity		
fossa		
foramen		
sulcus		
trochanter		
line		
crest		
condyle		
epicondyle		

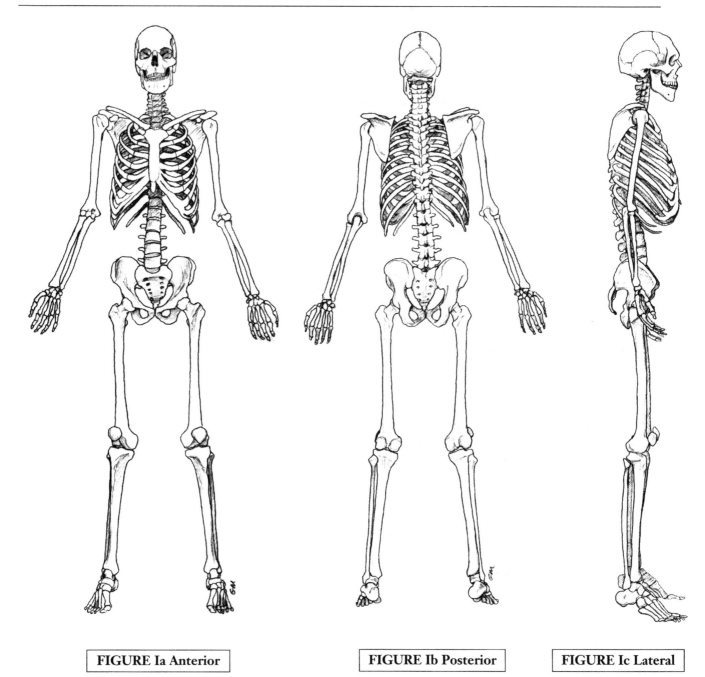

FIGURE Ia Anterior   **FIGURE Ib Posterior**   **FIGURE Ic Lateral**

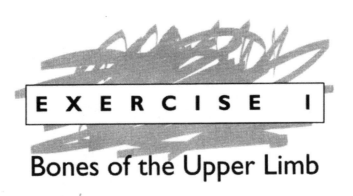

EXERCISE 1

Bones of the Upper Limb

THE PECTORAL GIRDLE

The illustrations on the facing page provide a view of the bones of the pectoral girdle: scapula and clavicle, with the humerus articulating with the scapula at the gleno-humeral joint. This girdle allows for the greatest movement of any joint in the human body; greatly due to the fact it is weakly 'jointed' to the axial skeleton. Note how these bones (the scapula posteriorly and the clavicle anteriorly) function as struts to anchor the upper limb to the thorax. The scapular attachment to the thorax is purely muscular and the muscles of the pectoral girdle function in maintaining structural integrity with the thorax. The scapula and clavicle also function together in positioning the humerus for the variety of activities it is involved in. The bones of the pectoral girdle are shown in FIGURES 1.1 and 1.2.

Before beginning specific study of the pectoral girdle outline the roughly triangular shape of the scapula in black on both the anterior and posterior views. In the anterior views do not color over the ribs. The **emphasis** here is that the anterior surface of the scapula lies along the posterior surface of ribs 2-7. (Color this surface yellow.)

The scapula is described as having superior, vertebral (near the vertebral column), and axillary (near the armpit) borders. The *superior border* (A) shows two prominent features: the *superior angle* (B) (where the superior and vertebral borders meet) and the *scapular notch* (C). Use your orange pencil to highlight the *superior border*. Highlight the *vertebral border* (D) with the yellow-green pencil and note how the *scapular spine* (E) arises from it. The *axillary border* (F) begins at the *inferior angle* (G), its junction with the vertebral border, and ends at the *glenoid fossa* (H). Highlight the axillary border in sky blue.

Fossas are depressions in bones and the scapula shows four of these: the aforementioned glenoid fossa is an integral part of the shoulder joint, accepting the head of the humerus (for details see next page). Just superior and in-

ferior to this fossa are small bumps, the *supraglenoid* (I) and *infraglenoid* (J) *tubercles*. The *supraspinous fossa* (K) is found on the posterior surface superior to the *scapular spine*; the *infraspinous fossa* (L) on the posterior surface below the scapular spine, and the *subscapular fossa* (M) on the anterior surface (see **emphasis** above)!

On the posterior view study the scapular spine and note how it flares out into a more flattened shape at its lateral end. This flattened portion is the *acromion process* (N); 'the tip of the shoulder'. It is from this landmark that a tailor measures the length of the upper limb in fitting a shirt or suit jacket.

The anterior side of the scapula also presents a prominence, the *coracoid process* (O), 'crow's beak'! The acromion process articulates with the lateral end of the clavicle to form the acromioclavicular joint. The seemingly unremarkable *clavicle* (P) provides the only articulation with the thorax via a joint with the sternum. It also serves as an important site of proximal or distal attachment of several important muscles. The slight *S* shape of this bone allows it to handle increased stress; even so the clavicle is the most frequently fractured bone in the body (broken 'collarbone'). Such an injury usually occurs in a fall on the outstretched hand accompanied by excessive application of an external force.

Two other injuries are common to the pectoral girdle: separation and dislocation. The first, usually called a shoulder separation, is misnamed, because the injury occurs between the distal end of the clavicle and the acromion; not at the shoulder. Separation of the acromioclavicular joint is often a consequence of falling on, or receiving a direct blow to, this joint.

A dislocation involves the head of the humerus (see next lesson) popping out of the muscular cuff surrounding it, and is therefore, an injury to the shoulder joint. This often occurs when the hand is supporting weight and a force acts upon the superior end of the humerus to move it anteriorly.

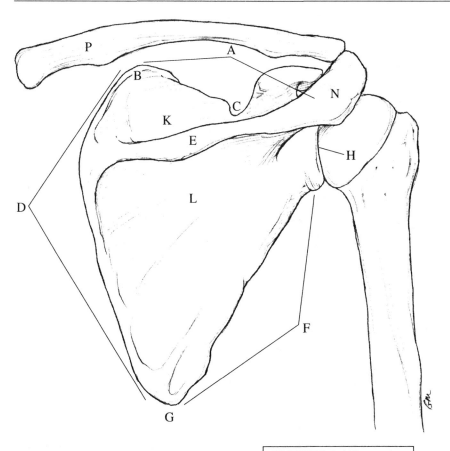
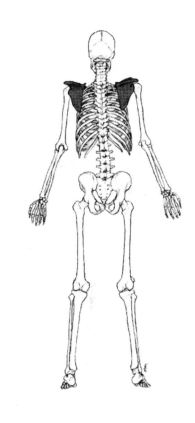

FIGURE 1.1 Posterior

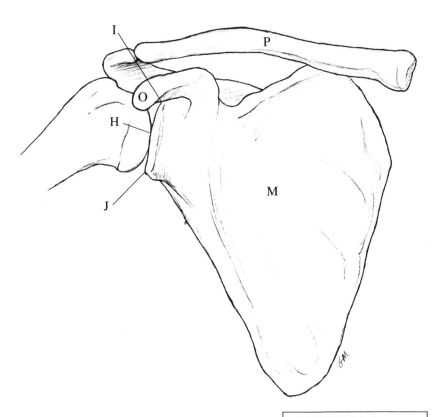
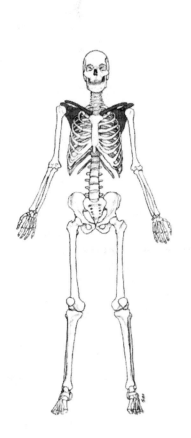

FIGURE 1.2 Anterior

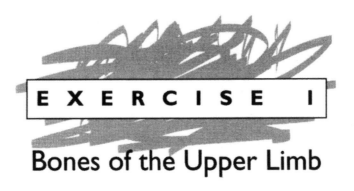

EXERCISE 1
Bones of the Upper Limb

THE ARM AND FOREARM

HUMERUS

For our purposes the arm is defined as the region of the upper limb between the shoulder and elbow, and the forearm the region between the elbow and wrist. The only bone of the arm is the humerus (color the identity bar red) (FIGURES 1.3 and 1.4). The most superior portion of the humerus, the *head* (A), is enlarged and smooth for articulation with the glenoid fossa (the glenohumeral joint; shoulder). Below the head of the humerus two 'necks' are commonly described The *anatomical neck* (B) forms a rim around the entire head and is the site of attachment of the fibrous capsule that encloses the glenohumeral joint. The surgical neck (C) is a descriptor of the area of the humerus where the enlarged 'head' gives way to the beginning of the shaft of the humerus, and where the bone is often fractured. Two important landmarks on the superior end of the humerus are the *greater* (D) and *lesser* (E) *tubercles*. In future work you will learn of muscles attaching to these tubercles. Between these tubercles lies a prominent depression, the *intertubercular groove* (F). The shaft (sometimes called the body) of the humerus is unremarkable except for a roughened swelling on the lateral surface at about mid-shaft; the *deltoid tuberosity* (G) and a slight *radial groove* (H) on the posterior surface.

The distal end of the humeral shaft flares out dramatically as the medial and lateral supracondylar ridges, which, in turn, become the *medial* (I) and *lateral* (J) *epicondyles*. These are important sites of muscle attachment. Two important adaptations of the distal end of the humerus are the *capitulum* (K) and *trochlea* (L). The trochlea forms a functional unit with the ulna (the elbow joint), while the capitulum forms a joint with the radius. Three fossae are found at the distal end of the humerus: anteriorly the *coronoid* (M) and *radial* (N) and posteriorly the *olecranon* (O). Each of these accepts the similarly named prominence of the bones of the forearm during flexion and extension at the elbow.

RADIUS AND ULNA

Two bones form the skeletal structure of the forearm: radius and ulna. Understand several things in FIGURES 1.3 and 1.4. The ulna is involved in flexion/extension at the elbow. The radius is involved in the movements of prona-

tion and supination of the forearm and hand. Note that the radius enlarges in thickness from proximal (elbow) to distal (wrist) while the ulna decreases in thickness. This is indicative of the role played by these bones in infrequent stress loading situations (handstands, tumbling routines, etc.), and very similar to the bones of the leg that routinely support weight. In life the gap between these bones is filled by an *interosseus membrane* which aids in transferring weight (stress) from the hand to the radius through the interosseus membrane, to the ulna, to the humerus, to the pectoral girdle, and hence to the thorax to be dissipated!

As with the humerus (and all long bones), the *radius* (identity bar: orange) and *ulna* (blue) are both described as having a body, or shaft, and a head. The *head of the radius* (P) articulates with the capitulum of the humerus and the *radial notch of the ulna*. Inferior to the head lies the neck of the radius (Q) and a prominent swelling, the *radial tuberosity* (R), for distal attachment of the powerful biceps brachii muscle. The body (shaft) of the radius is unremarkable except at its distal end where it enlarges to an *articular surface* (S) for union with the carpal bones, an articular surface with the ulna (*the ulnar notch*, T), and a pointed projection, *the styloid process* (U). The distal end of the radius is particularly susceptible to fracture, often from a fall on the outstretched hand (Colles' fracture).

The proximal end of the posterior surface of the ulna is distinguished by the *olecranon process* (V) for distal attachment of the powerful triceps brachii muscle. Anteriorly the *coronoid process* (W) is found, with a roughened area, the *ulnar tuberosity* (X), for distal attachment of the brachialis muscle. Between these two processes lies the deep *trochlear notch* (Y) for articulation with the humerus. The proximal end of the body (shaft) of the ulna features a *radial notch* (Y_1) for articulation with the *head of the radius*. The distal end of the ulna is called the *head* (Z) and exhibits two features: an *articular surface with the radius* (T_1) and a *styloid process* (U_1).

❓ FOR REVIEW AND THOUGHT

Dislocation is a common problem for the glenohumeral (shoulder) joint but seldom occurs at the humeroulnar (elbow) joint. Why?

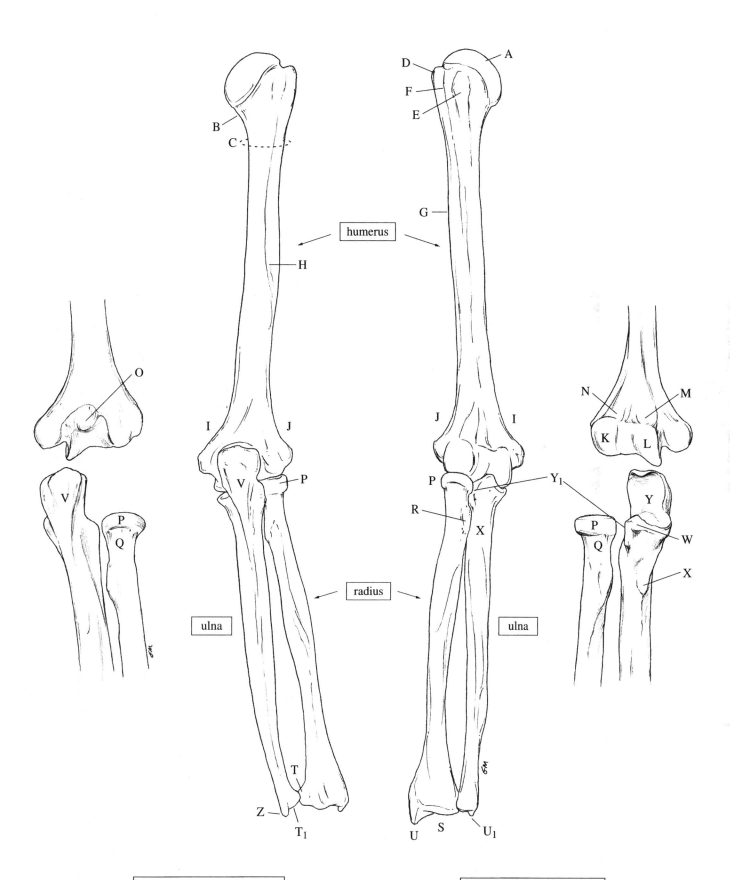

FIGURE 1.3 Posterior

FIGURE 1.4 Anterior

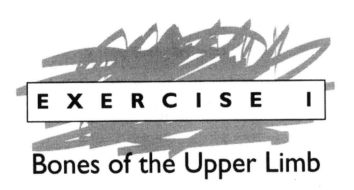

EXERCISE 1

Bones of the Upper Limb

THE WRIST AND HAND

The most 'functionally significant' portion of the upper limb is that of the wrist and hand. In some sense it truly may be said that the remainder of the upper limb serves only to position the hand. In using this text: turning the pages, coloring, and note taking, you are constantly and finely positioning your wrist, hand, and individual fingers. As you read this the great muscles of the arm, buttocks, and thigh are playing very little role. (Your buttocks may be getting tired but it is not due to powerful muscular contraction.)

The bones of the wrist and hand are nicely organized for learning and appreciation. Let us first study the carpals. These eight bones are arranged in two concave rows. Anatomical convention describes these bones (and those of the metacarpals and phalanges) from lateral to medial in the anatomical position. Review the anatomical position (FIGURE Intro.1) then place your hands on the desk in front of you, palms up, to appreciate what you see in FIGURE 1.5. This position of the hands is called *supination*. Now turn them palms down to understand FIGURE 1.6. This position is called *pronation*.

CARPALS

The proximal row of carpals:

Scaphoid (Navicular) (A) (color yellow)
Lunate (B) (color orange)
Triquetral (Triquetrum) (C) (color red-orange)
Pisiform (D) (color red)

The distal row of carpals:

Trapezium (E) (color yellow-green)
Trapeziod (F) (color green)
Capitate (G) (color sky blue)
Hamate (H) (color blue)

Several of these bones require further explanation and study. In the proximal row the *scaphoid (sometimes called navicular because of a fancied resemblance to a boat)* is the main carpal articulating with the distal end of the radius. When you take your pulse you do so by pressing the wall of the radial artery against the hard surface of this bone.

The *pisiform* is very superficial and is often bruised in childhood falls. Find the pisiform in your right wrist in the pad at the base of your fifth digit. It is the bony prominence just distal to the crease separating your forearm from your hand. Push on this hard enough to feel a bit of dull pain.

In the distal row of carpals find the *trapezium* articulating with the first metacarpal. Study the surfaces of the trapezium involved in this articulation. What do you see? This joint is described as a saddle joint; does this make sense given what you have just seen?

In the distal row also find the *hamate* and note the prominence, or hook, it presents. The hook of the hamate and the pisiform are landmarks for the passage of an important nerve into the hand (ulnar nerve). These bony landmarks (medially) and the scaphoid and trapezium (laterally) form the boundaries of a tunnel roofed by fibrous connective tissue. Through this 'carpal tunnel' pass nine tendons and another major nerve (median nerve) to the hand.

METACARPALS

The *metacarpals* are numbered 1 through 5 from lateral to medial (again see the anatomical position). Each has a proximal base, a shaft, and a distal head. The metacarpals provide the 'bulk' of the hand. Color the metacarpals violet.

PHALANGES

The *phalanges* are numbered as are the metacarpals. Digit 1 has only two phalanges (proximal and distal; phalanx, singular), whereas digits 2-5 have proximal, middle, and distal phalanges. On each of the digits color the phalanges in this way: proximal (light brown), middle (brown), distal (black).

❓ FOR REVIEW AND THOUGHT

Review the bones involved in the joints of the upper limb. What movements are allowed at each joint? (refer to Introduction: A Beginning (p.1) and the discussion of planes and axes.) Are these movements related to the size or shape of the bones involved?

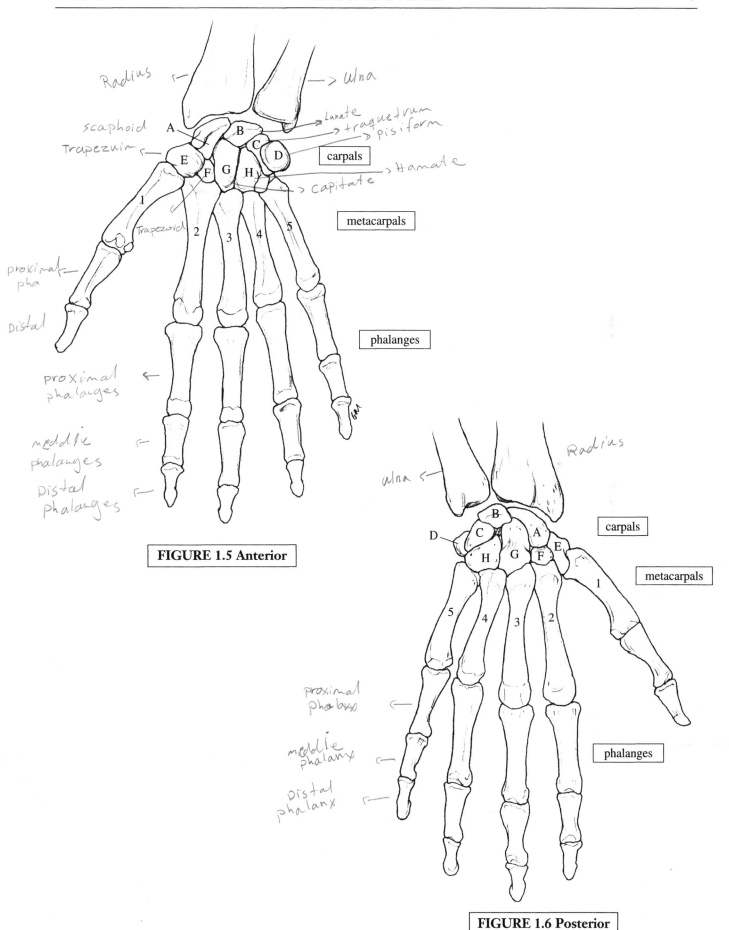

Radius

Ulna

scaphoid

A

B

C

D

Lunate

traquetrum

pisiform

carpals

Trapezuin

E

F

G

H

Hamate

capitate

metacarpals

1

Trapezoid

2

3

4

5

proximal pha

Distal

proximal phalanges

phalanges

meddie phalanges

Distal phalanges

FIGURE 1.5 Anterior

ulna

Radius

B

D

C

A

E

H

G

F

carpals

metacarpals

1

5

4

3

2

proximal phalano

meddie phalanx

Distal phalanx

phalanges

FIGURE 1.6 Posterior

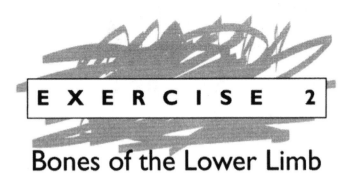

Bones of the Lower Limb

THE PELVIC GIRDLE

As you progress through this section of the skeletal system make notes on similarities and differences between the upper and lower limbs. Ask yourself (or a partner) why such similarities or differences exist. If you keep in mind a common 'system of arrangement' between the upper and lower limbs you will reduce the need for memory work, and replace it with understanding.

Prior to beginning your study of the pelvic girdle return to the illustration of the entire skeleton and note the anterior tilt of the pelvis. This is normal! The pelvis does not lie horizontal, rather as a consequence of the human upright stance it presents itself as if to allow a view of the abdomen.

Each half of the pelvic girdle (os coxae) is composed of three developmentally separate bones; the ilium, ischium, and pubis, all joining in the *acetabulum* (A) (L., vinegar cup), the deep cavity on the lateral aspect. Identify the approximate extent of each on FIGURE 2.1. The *ilium* is the most superior portion of the pelvic girdle, forming the superior portion of the acetabulum and the wing (ala) rising and spreading from the main structure. The *ischium* forms the posteroinferior portion of the acetabulum and the posterior portion of the coxal bone. The *pubis* forms the anterior portion of the acetabulum and the anteromedial portion of the coxal structure. The approximate boundaries of these three bones are shown in hatched lines. Outline the *ilium* in red, the *ischium* in blue, and the *pubis* in yellow; and color their identity bars in the same manner! Having done so let's identify specific landmark structures on the pelvic girdle.

ILIUM

The ilium (FIGURES 2.2, 2.3) shows several important landmarks. The rim of the wing is the *iliac crest* (B) and the internal surface is the *iliac fossa* (C). The iliac crest itself has several important landmarks; most posterior is the *iliac tuberosity* (D) with *posterior superior* (E) and *posterior inferior* (F) *iliac spines*. Anteriorly the iliac crest is distinguished by the *anterior superior iliac spine* (G) and the *anterior inferior iliac spine* (H). Along its lateral surface the ilium displays *inferior* (I_1), *anterior* (I_2), and *posterior* (I_3) *gluteal lines*; evidence of the attachments of the gluteal muscles. Use your red pencil to underline each of these landmarks.

ISCHIUM

The ischium (FIGURES 2.2, 2.3) is composed of a body and a ramus (L., branch). Identify the *body* (J) and the *ramus* (K). A prominent bump on the ramus is the *ischial tuberosity* (L). If you are sitting while doing this lesson you are balancing on the ischial tuberosities. The uncomfortable feeling that comes from sitting on a hard bench or chair for a long period of time is due to this fact. The pointed posteromedial projection from the ramus is the *ischial spine* (M). This spine demarcates the greater sciatic notch (superior) and lesser sciatic notch (inferior). Use your blue pencil to underline each of these landmarks.

PUBIS

Each pubic bone (FIGURES 2.2, 2.3) resembles a V turned sideways. The *body* (N) articulates with its contralateral counterpart at the pubic symphysis. Two rami emanate from the body. The *superior ramus* (O) is distinguished by the *pubic tubercle* (P) and the *pubic crest* (Q); both serving as sites of muscle attachment. The *inferior ramus* (R) unites with the ischial ramus. Use your yellow pencil to underline each of these landmarks.

▶ ACTIVE LEARNING

Using a skeletal specimen find the large obturator foramen immediately inferior to the acetabulum. This 'hole' was not discussed on this page because in life it does not exist in this state. It is 90-95% covered with a membrane and internal and external muscles.

❓ FOR REVIEW AND THOUGHT

Unlike the fragile connection of the pectoral girdle to the sternum and thorax the pelvic girdle is securely fastened to the sacral portion of the vertebral column. Why these differences? What are the positives and negatives of such differences at each joint? While the basic concept of each joint is the same why does one have a much deeper 'cup' for articulation with a limb than the other? What implications does this have for joint function?

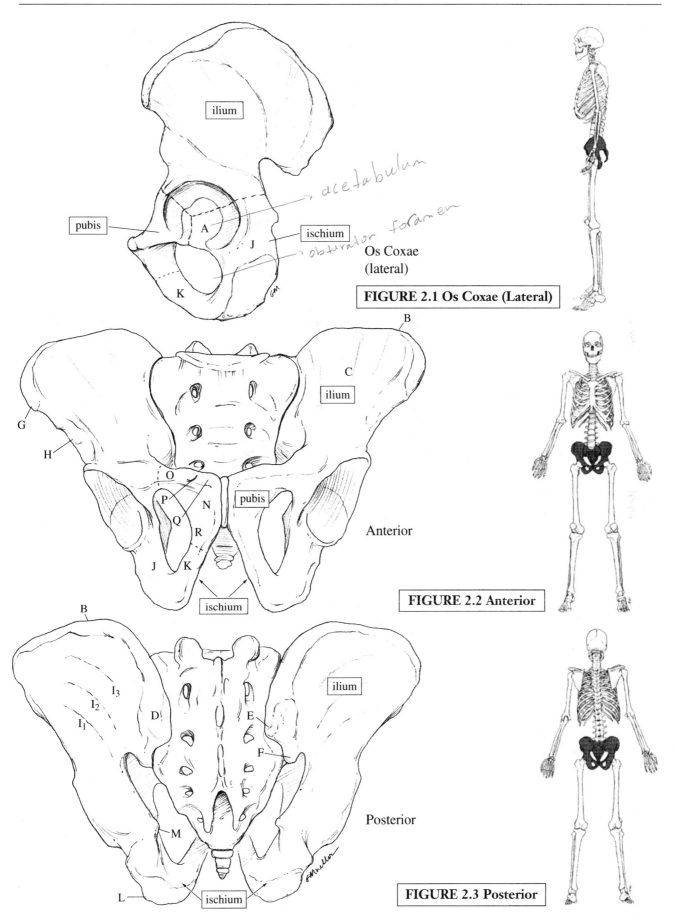

ilium

acetabulum

pubis

obturator foramen

A

ischium

J

K

Os Coxae
(lateral)

FIGURE 2.1 Os Coxae (Lateral)

B

C

ilium

G

H

O

P

N

pubis

Q

R

J

K

ischium

Anterior

FIGURE 2.2 Anterior

B

I_3

I_2

I_1

D

E

F

ilium

M

Posterior

L

ischium

FIGURE 2.3 Posterior

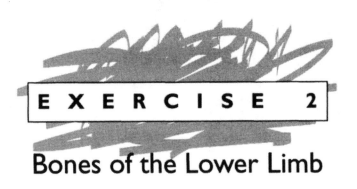

EXERCISE 2

Bones of the Lower Limb

MALE/FEMALE PELVIS

Compare and contrast the pelves in FIGURE 2.4a-d. The key comparisons should be made with the *ischial spines* (A) and the degree to which they protrude into the pelvic bowl and the *subpubic angle* (B) presented by the inferior pubic rami.

The female pelvis differs from the male for one reason: childbirth! The entrance to the pelvis is the *superior aperture* (C) and the exit the *inferior aperture* (D). The head of the fetus must negotiate its way through the pelvis via these apertures. The word pelvis derives from the Greek word **pyelos:** *an oblong trough!* The relative ease or difficulty of passage through this trough is dependent upon its transverse and anteroposterior dimensions.

Humans show a variety of pelvic structures but three general forms are most frequent. The *anthropoid pelvis* is found in a few males and in about 23% of all females. In this pelvis the anteroposterior dimension of the superior aperture is greater than the transverse diameter. This form also has prominent ischial spines and a narrow subpubic angle.

The *android pelvis* is easily the most common in males and is also seen in approximately 33% of females. This form shows prominent *ischial spines* and a narrow *subpubic angle* defined by the pubic rami. A view of the superior pelvic aperture appears heart-shaped.

The most common pelvic form in women (42%) is *gynecoid*. The contrast of its roominess to the two forms previously studied is obvious. This pelvis shows a wide pubic arch and ischial spines that do not protrude medially as greatly. A superior view shows a rounded and open aperture.

If you have added the percentages of these three pelvic types, you have reached only 98%. Two percent of women show a *platypelloid* pelvis—especially narrow anteroposteriorly and wide transversely. The opening of the superior aperture is diminished making delivery more difficult. This pelvic structure is more often associated with the need for cesarean section than the other forms.

❓ FOR REVIEW AND THOUGHT

The wider girth of the female pelvis has implications at the knee. Due to the increased angle at which the femur meets the tibia the knee joint is somewhat less stable in women. What implications does this have for girls and women preparing for athletic participation?

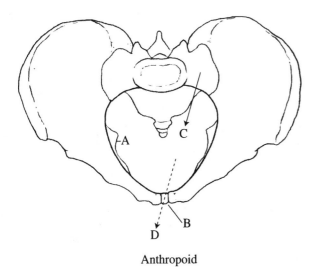

Anthropoid

FIGURE 2.4a Anthropoid

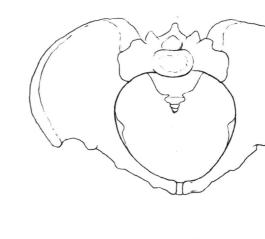

Android

FIGURE 2.4b Android

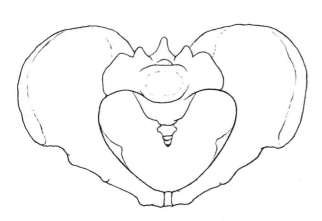

Gynecoid

FIGURE 2.4c Gynecoid

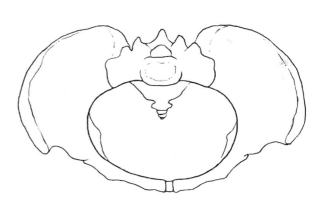

Platypelloid

FIGURE 2.4d Platypelloid

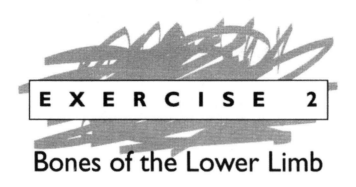

EXERCISE 2

Bones of the Lower Limb

THE THIGH AND LEG

FEMUR

For our purposes the thigh is defined as the region of the lower limb between the hip and the knee, and the leg as the region between the knee and ankle (FIGURES 2.5 and 2.6). The most readily identifiable structure is the massive femur; the only bone of the thigh (color its identity bar green). At its superior end the *head* (A) fits snugly into the acetabulum of the ox coxae. The *neck* (B) of the femur is angled approximately 45^0 from the *shaft* (C). At the point where the neck and shaft meet two prominent landmarks are found: the *greater* (D) and *lesser* (E) *trochanters*. Anteriorly the trochanters are connected by an *intertrochanteric line* (F), while posteriorly the connection is more pronounced as the *intertrochanteric crest* (G). These form a rim around the base of the femoral neck and are the site of attachment of the fibrous capsule enclosing the coxofemoral joint. On the posterolateral surface of the femur, somewhat inferior to the greater trochanter you will find a roughened area, the *gluteal tuberosity* (H), the distal attachment of the powerful gluteus maximus, continued inferiorly as the *gluteal line*. Just inferior to the lesser trochanter you will find the *pectineal line* (I), also the site of attachment of a muscle you will learn in a future lesson. Please note how these two lines: *gluteal and pectineal*, converge to form a ridge coursing most of the length of the posterior surface of the shaft of the femur. This ridge is the *linea aspera* (J). Also note that the linea aspera represents the midline of the femur! (Color the linea aspera orange.)

The linea aspera ends by diverging into *supracondylar ridges* leading to the *lateral* (L) and *medial* (M) *condyles*. The ridge to the medial condyle is somewhat more pronounced and at its termination shows a small bump, the *adductor tubercle* (N). Both condyles present an articular surface for union with the tibia. An *intercondylar fossa* (O) and *patellar articular surface* (P) are also present.

TIBIA AND FIBULA

Two bones form the skeletal framework of the leg: the tibia and fibula. The size difference between the two is readily apparent and has its basis on the amount of weight borne by each bone. Note that only the tibia participates in the knee joint. Both the tibia and fibula, however, play important roles in the structure and stability of the ankle joint. In life a strong interosseus membrane connects these two bones and aids in transferring forces between them.

A prominent *tuberosity* (Q) is the most obvious landmark on the tibia (color bar: yellow); found anteriorly just inferior to the knee joint. The proximal end of the tibia also expands slightly into *medial* (R) and *lateral* (S) *condyles*; articulating with their femoral counterparts. A slight projection, the *intercondylar eminence* (T) is also found. The shaft of the tibia remains very constant in shape and diameter throughout its length and presents a prominent anterior edge in its distal two thirds (the shinbone); something all of us have bruised at one time or another. On the posterior surface find the *soleal line* (U), another landmark of muscle attachment.

At the distal end of the medial side of the tibia find the *medial malleolus* (V), an important component of the structural integrity of the ankle joint. On the posterior surface of the medial malleolus is a *groove* (W) caused by the tendon of the tibialis posterior muscle as it passes into the foot. A final landmark, on the lateral surface, is the *fibular notch* (X), for the distal articulation with the fibula.

The fibula (color bar: blue) is an unremarkable bone, serving only slightly in weight bearing. Like the tibia it is very constant in shape and diameter throughout its length. The fibula's role is mainly that of a site of muscle attachment; most importantly for muscles passing into the foot. Only three landmarks are described for the fibula: the *head* (Y), articulating superiorly with the lateral condyle of the tibia; the *shaft* (Z); and the prominent inferior end, the *lateral malleolus* (Z_1); an important player in ankle stability.

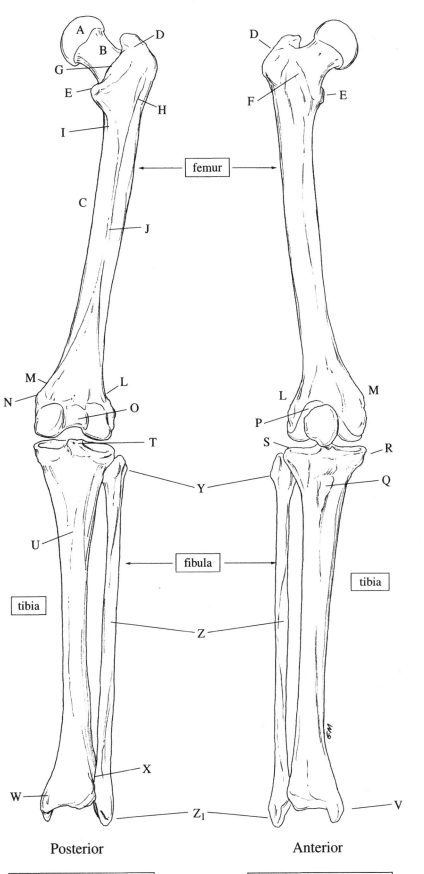

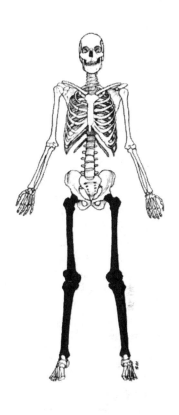

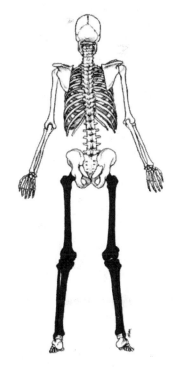

Posterior

Anterior

FIGURE 2.5 Posterior

FIGURE 2.6 Anterior

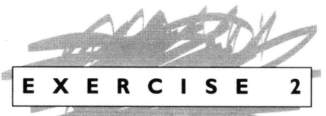

EXERCISE 2
Bones of the Lower Limb

THE FOOT

Standing on your own two feet is a maxim of our society implying independence and integrity. The statement derives from the fact that as a child of about one year of age you literally gained a great deal of independence when the bones and muscles of your lower limbs acquired sufficient strength; allowing you to begin upright locomotion. Previously you were asked to place your hands on the desk in front of you to aid in understanding the structure of the hand. Please do so again, with palms down. This mimics the permanent position of your feet! Now, take your shoes and socks off! This leads to the introduction of two new terms: plantar (the inferior surface of the foot; in lay language, the sole); and dorsum (the superior surface of the foot). The physical organization of the bones of the foot is not quite as clear as that of the hand; nonetheless let's forge ahead!

TARSALS

Seven bones form the core of the foot (FIGURES 2.7, 2.8, and 2.9). Two, the calcaneus (color orange) and talus (color green), are critical for maintenance of ankle and foot integrity and stability. The *calcaneus* (A) provides the base of support for the posterior of the foot. The powerful gastrocnemius and soleus muscles have their distal attachment on the posterior surface of the calcaneus. The plantar surface of the calcaneus presents the *tuber calcanei* (A_1). On the superomedial aspect of the calcaneus find the *sustentaculum tali* (A_2). This projection of the calcaneus literally aids in 'sustaining' (supporting) the talus! The calcaneus also shows a deep groove on its inferior surface; formed by the tendon of the flexor hallucis longus muscle (A_3).

The bone most functionally related to the calcaneus is the *talus* (B). The talus is described as having a *head* (B_1), a *neck* (B_2), and a *body* (B_3). The talus sits atop the calcaneus and is wedged tightly between the medial and lateral malleoli (see previous lesson). This portion of the talus is the *trochlea tali* (B_4). This union, structurally sound by virtue of the manner in which the trochlea tali (pulley) is positioned, is further strengthened by ligaments on both the medial and lateral sides.

Anterior to the talus find the *navicular* (C) (color blue) with a roughened tuberosity (C_1) on its inferomedial surface. Anterior to the calcaneus is the *cuboid* (D) (color yellow). Observe the nearly 'transverse tarsal joint' between these four bones. This is not a joint anatomically; but functionally it allows slight movement within the foot as well as inversion and eversion of the foot. Such movements are important in balance activities and locomotion on uneven ground. The cuboid exhibits a deep groove on its plantar surface (D_1) caused by the *tendon of the peroneus*

longus muscle. The remaining three tarsals are the *medial* (E), *intermediate* (F), and *lateral* (G) *cuneiform bones*. (Color all three brown.)

METATARSALS

As with the hand, the foot has five metatarsals numbered 1-5 from medial to lateral. Each has a proximal base, a shaft, and a distal head. A prominent *tuberosity* is found on the lateral surface of the base of the fifth metatarsal (H). This tuberosity is the site of attachment of the peroneus brevis muscle, but you encounter it more in sizing the width of shoes. Color the metatarsals violet.

PHALANGES

These are numbered as are the metatarsals. The pattern is the same as in the hand. The great toe is similar to the thumb in having only two phalanges (proximal and distal) and the remaining digits each have three: proximal, middle, and distal. Color the phalanges black.

❓ FOR REVIEW AND THOUGHT

Compare 'equivalent' joints of the lower and upper limbs: hip and shoulder, knee and elbow, ankle and wrist, metacarpals/metatarsals, and phalanges. Which movements are similar, which different? Why? What are the enhancing or limiting factors?

☾ JUST FOR FUN

Wolff's Law states that a bone develops the structure most suited to resist forces acting upon it (a 'use it or lose it' concept). Load placed upon bone leads to growth, and lack of load (as in long-term bedridden patients or astronauts in a weightless environment) leads to bone loss. One load every human bears is weight. In normal posture a human bears weight equally on each foot. Within each foot the calcaneus and the heads of the metatarsals each bear half the load, distributed in this manner: six units on the tuber calcanei, two units on the head of the first metatarsal, and one unit on each of the remaining four metatarsal heads. Verify this by noting that the first metatarsal is about twice the thickness of the other four, and that these four are almost exactly the same thickness. Calculate the weight distribution on the calcanei and metatarsals of a 120 lb. human standing still with weight equally balanced on both feet! Your answer?

After doing this keep in mind that humans rarely spend any time standing still, equally balanced, on both feet!

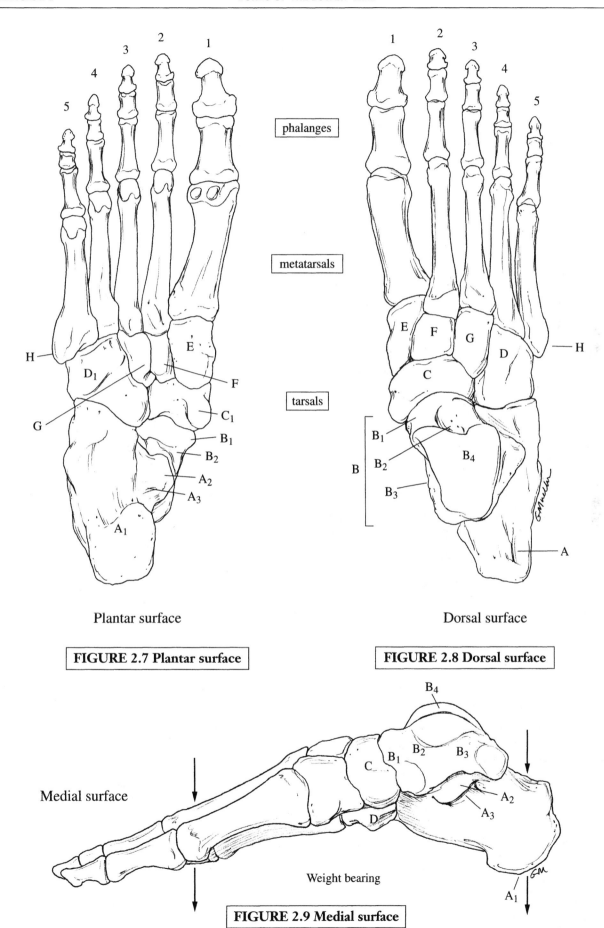

phalanges

metatarsals

tarsals

Plantar surface

Dorsal surface

FIGURE 2.7 Plantar surface

FIGURE 2.8 Dorsal surface

Medial surface

Weight bearing

FIGURE 2.9 Medial surface

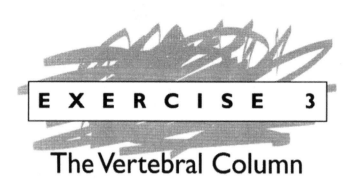

EXERCISE 3

The Vertebral Column

Before studying individual vertebrae or regions become familiar with the entire vertebral column (FIGURES 3.1a and 3.1b). The vertebral column (spine; spinal column) is the core structural and support unit of the trunk, plays a key role in movement and the upright stance, and protects the spinal cord. The human column typically consists of 33 vertebrae: 7 cervical; 12 thoracic; 5 lumbar; 5 sacral (fused to form the sacrum); and 4 coccygeal (of which the first is sometimes separate and the remaining three fused).

Ligamentous and cartilagenous structures aid in maintaining stability, and limiting mobility, of the vertebral column (FIGURE 3.1c). An intimately vital constituent of this 'stack of separate bones' is the series of fibrocartilagenous *intervertebral disks* uniting succeeding vertebral bodies from the second cervical vertebra to the lumbosacral junction! The disks also serve as cushions, preserving vertebral integrity during weight-bearing activities (walking, running, jumping). Each disk has a core of gelatinous material, the *nucleus pulposus* (color orange), surrounded by a wrapping of elastic and fibrous connective tissue, the *annulus fibrosus* (color red). Sometimes this core tries to break out of its fibrous ring: a ruptured or herniated disk. This is most common in the lumbar region and often results in significant pain due to impingement on nerves to the lower limb.

Four ligaments are also associated with the vertebral column; functioning to maintain integrity of the column and limit movement. The *anterior longitudinal ligament* (A) (color yellow) courses along the anterior surface of the vertebral bodies. The *posterior longitudinal ligament* (B) (color green) is found running the length of the column on the posterior surface of the vertebral bodies. The *ligamentum flavum* (C) (color brown) is actually a repetitive series passing from one vertebra to another on the deep surface of the laminae. The *supraspinous ligament* (D) (color blue) passes along the spinous processes of the vertebrae, and also sends slips into the gaps between individual spinous processes; the *interspinous ligaments* (E) (color violet). In the neck the supraspinous ligament is thickened as the *ligamentum nuchae* (F), which functions in holding up (stabilizing) the head. This structure is very powerful and vital in quadraped creatures and is functionally continuous with the supraspinous ligament. (Picture in your mind the cow grazing in a field or two rams butting one another and lifting their pelvis and hind limbs in reaction.)

🌀 JUST FOR FUN

Let's create a concept for learning and understanding the structure of an individual vertebra. The concept is of a church building and how the structural elements of this building represent structural components of a vertebra. The sizes or shapes of the constituent parts may vary (not all churches are constructed exactly the same) but the concept will remain true!

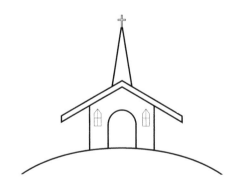

Color the ground brown, the walls blue, the roof yellow, the gable green, and the steeple orange. The simile we are constructing is as follows.

Ground	=	vertebral body	=	brown
Walls	=	pedicle	=	blue
Roof	=	lamina	=	yellow
Gable	=	transverse process	=	green
Steeple	=	spinous process	=	orange

Use this coloring scheme throughout your study of the vertebrae.

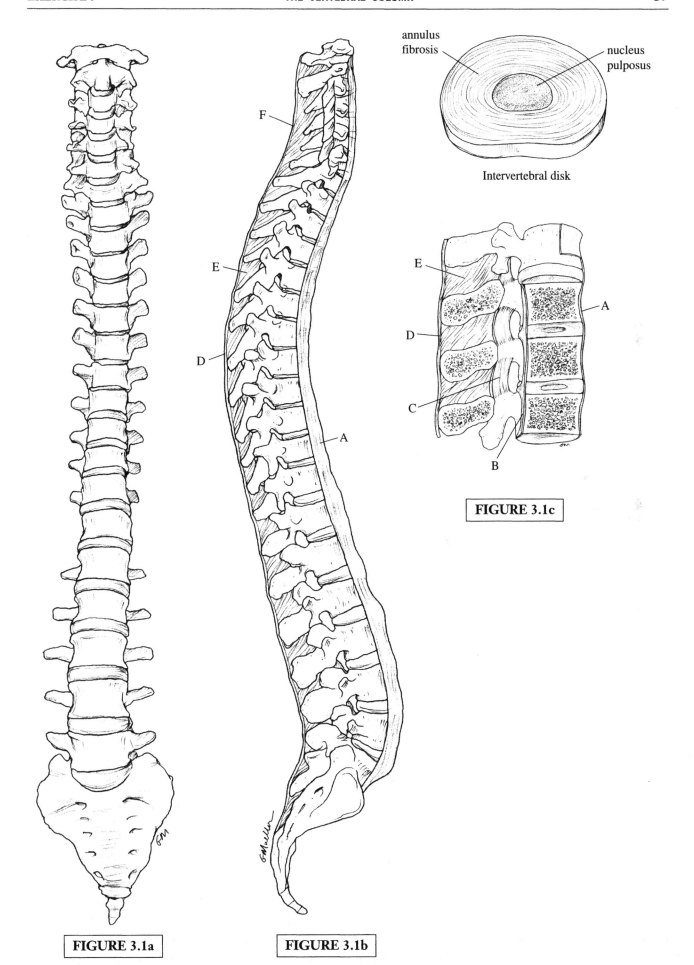

annulus
fibrosis

nucleus
pulposus

Intervertebral disk

FIGURE 3.1c

FIGURE 3.1a   **FIGURE 3.1b**

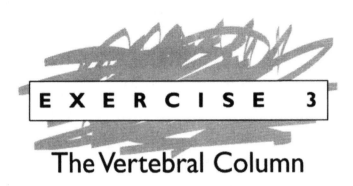

EXERCISE 3

The Vertebral Column

The vertebral column presents several anteroposterior curves. The cervical and lumbar curves are concave posteriorly and are described as acquired. These curves develop as a natural consequence of the human upright stance. The cervical curve begins to form as a baby lifts its head and, in concert with the lumbar curve, continues to define itself via other stages in assuming the biped position (crawling, walking). The thoracic and sacral curves are concave anteriorly and described as congenital (present at birth). In the upright position these gentle curves serve to balance the body over its center of gravity. An exaggeration of a congenital curve is called a *kyphosis* (most common in the thoracic region) (FIGURE 3.1d) and an exaggeration of an acquired curve is called a *lordosis* (most common in the lumbar region) (FIGURE 3.1e).

The vertebral column also adapts to maintain itself against the force of gravity in a right/left fashion. Deviation of one portion of the column to one side is usually accompanied by a compensating deviation to the opposite side in another part of the column. Such lateral deviation is *scoliosis* (FIGURE 3.1f). Nearly all of us have some slight functional scoliosis due to the fact that we are 'handed' and tend to do most things (carry book bags, briefcases, babes in arms, etc.) with a favored limb. Structural scoliosis is quite another matter and may include a twisting of the thoracic cage and resulting 'hump back'.

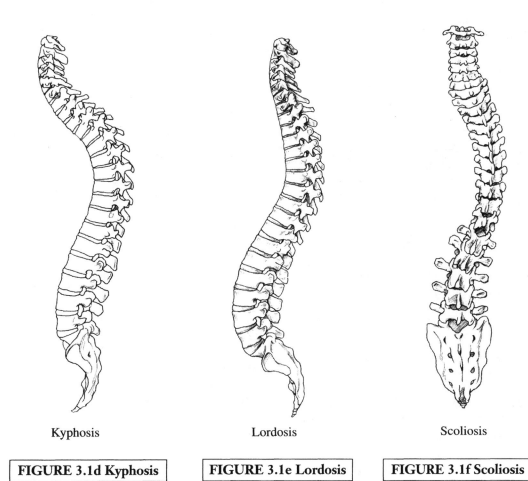

Kyphosis   Lordosis   Scoliosis

FIGURE 3.1d Kyphosis   **FIGURE 3.1e Lordosis**   **FIGURE 3.1f Scoliosis**

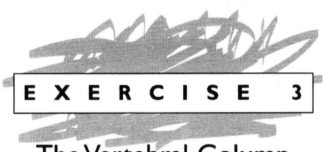

EXERCISE 3

The Vertebral Column

CERVICAL REGION

The structure of typical cervical vertebra (FIGURE 3.2) (color bar yellow) includes a *body* (A), and a *vertebral arch* (B) with its component portions: *pedicle* (C), and *lamina* (D) surrounding the *vertebral foramen* (E). (All of this to protect the spinal cord which passes through the sequential vertebral foramina.) A prominent *spinous process* (F) is formed at the junction of the laminae and *transverse processes* (G) are shown at the junction of the laminae and pedicles. Each vertebra has *superior* (H) and *inferior* (I) *articular processes* with smooth *facets* for articulation with superior and inferior vertebrae. Each transverse process shows *anterior* (J) and *posterior* (K) *tubercles* as well as a *transverse foramen* (L). Note: the vertebral artery makes its way to the head via the channel formed by the sequential transverse foramina. This journey begins at C_6 vertebral level; therefore C_7 vertebrae lack these foramina.

The cervical region also presents two very 'untypical' vertebrae: the atlas and axis (FIGURES 3.3 and 3.4). Look at these illustrations briefly, then return to the conceptualized church/vertebra and attempt to determine which structural components are altered or missing!

The first cervical vertebra, the *axis* (FIGURE 3.3), is so named because it holds up the head, as the mythical Greek strongman Atlas held up the world. This vertebra lacks a body; being structured as two arches. The *anterior arch* (M) shows a slight depression on its internal surface, the *fovea dentis* (N). The *posterior arch* (O) has no particular distinguishing characteristics. The two arches meet bilaterally to form a *lateral mass* (P) with superior and inferior articular facets. Transverse processes extend from the lateral mass and surround the transverse foramen. On the posterior surface of the superior articular facet is a deep groove. This is the *sulcus for the vertebral artery* (Q). After ascending through the transverse foramina of the cervical vertebrae the artery curves sharply posteriorly and enters the skull through the foramen magnum.

The second cervical vertebra, the *axis* (axis: core, center of rotation) (FIGURE 3.4) has an extra body (the body that the atlas lost in embryologic development). This is the *dens, or odontoid process* (R). This process articulates superiorly with the *fovea dentis;* held tightly in place by a strong ligament. This arrangement allows rotation of the skull on the neck! Other features of the axis include those of other cervical vertebrae. A *vertebral arch* (S), *transverse processes* with foramina (T), *vertebral foramen* (U), *superior* (V) and *inferior* (W) *articular processes and facets.*

THORACIC REGION

Thoracic vertebrae are unique in their extremely pointed, and overlapping, spinous processes and their special articulations with the ribs. FIGURE 3.5 (color bar red) provides superior and lateral views of a thoracic vertebra.

The *body* (A) shows *superior* (B) and *inferior* (C) *costal facets* for articulation with its rib and a partial articulation with the rib below. A *vertebral arch* (D) with *laminar* (E) and *pedicular* (F) components is present. At the junction of lamina and pedicle are *superior* (G) and *inferior facets* (H) for articulation with the vertebrae immediately superior and inferior. The pedicle shows a shallow notch on its superior surface and a significantly deeper notch inferiorly. A prominent and inferiorly directed *spinous process* (I) is obvious. The *transverse processes* (J) extend laterally and show *facets* (K) for articulation with corresponding ribs.

LUMBAR REGION

Lumbar vertebrae (FIGURE 3.6) (color bar blue) are characterized by their large size, and massive spinous and transverse processes. The *body* (L) is impressive in its size. The *vertebral arch* (M) with *pedicles* (N) and *laminae* (O) also presents an impression of sturdiness. Like thoracic vertebrae, the pedicles of lumbar vertebrae also show small superior and large inferior notches. Since lumbar vertebrae do not articulate with ribs their *transverse processes* (P) serve as sites of attachment of powerful muscles. *Superior* (Q) and *inferior* (R) *articular processes with facets* are found extending from the vertebral arch for articulation with the vertebrae immediately superior and inferior. Note the difference in size and orientation of the *spinous process* (S) in comparison to thoracic vertebrae.

❓ FOR REVIEW AND THOUGHT

We have finished study of the individual vertebra. Study a completely articulated vertebral column to aid in answering these questions. Observe the size of the vertebral bodies from the first cervical to the fifth lumbar. Observe the directional orientation of the vertebral facets from the first cervical to the fifth lumbar. What do these observations imply in regard to the various functions of the vertebral column described at the beginning of our study? What is the reason for the superior and inferior vertebral notches of successive vertebrae?

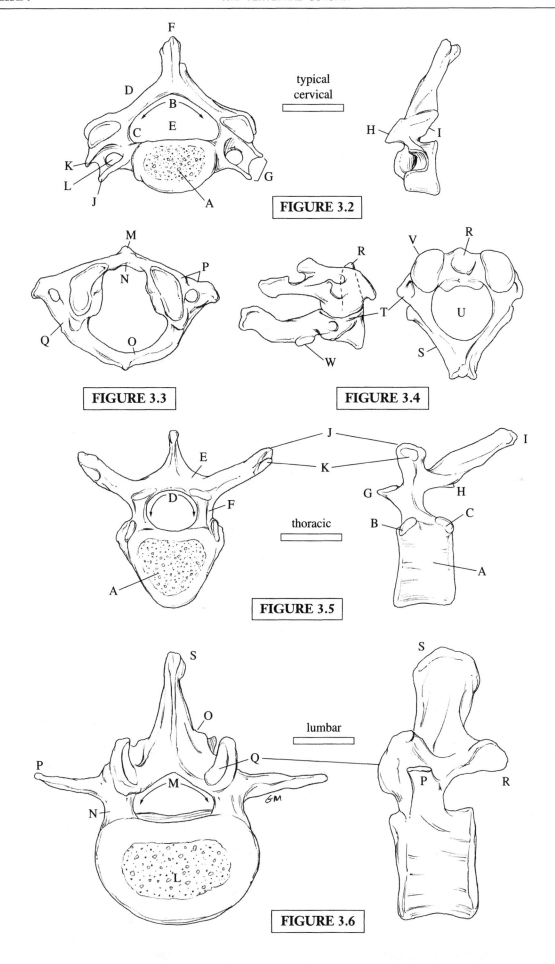

typical
cervical

FIGURE 3.2

FIGURE 3.3

FIGURE 3.4

thoracic

FIGURE 3.5

lumbar

FIGURE 3.6

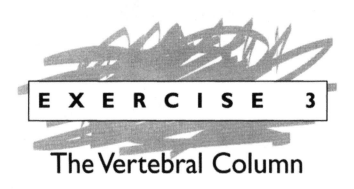

EXERCISE 3

The Vertebral Column

SACRUM

The massive sacrum, wedged tightly between the ilia (the sacroiliac joints), represents five fused sacral vertebrae. From earlier work you know that the sacral curve is congenital and concave. The sacrum (FIGURES 3.7a,b) articulates superiorly with the fifth lumbar vertebra, a joint critical for the stability of the vertebral column and the point of greatest change in curvature in the entire column. It presents *superior articular facets* (A) for this union.

On its posterior (dorsal) surface the sacrum shows a series of vestigial remnants of individual vertebra. The *median sacral crest* (B) represents fused spinous processes, the *intermediate sacral crests* (C) are the remains of articular processes, and the *lateral sacral crests* (D) of transverse processes. On this surface also find bilateral *sacral tuberosities* (E). Lateral to each tuberosity is the *auricular surface* (F) for junction with the corresponding ilium at the sacroiliac joint. Four pairs of *dorsal foramina* (G) are also seen.

The *sacral canal* (H) and the *sacral hiatus* (I) are also seen posteriorly. Projecting inferiorly on the right and left of the hiatus is the *sacral cornu* (J). The inferior tip of the sacrum is the *apex* (K) and the superior tip is the *base* (L).

On its anterior (ventral, pelvic) surface the sacrum may show *transverse lines* (M) indicating the lines of fusion of the five sacral vertebrae. The anterior aspect of the base is particularly prominent: the *sacral promontory* (N). Four pairs of *ventral foramina* (O) are present.

COCCYX

The coccyx is the vestigial remnant of four separate vertebrae. Its only notable landmark is the *cornu* (P).

❓ FOR REVIEW AND THOUGHT

How did the various structural components of the vertebrae (spinous processes, articular facets, transverse processes, pedicles, laminae, and bodies) change in the various regions?

What are the developmental and functional reasons for the structure of the various vertebrae?

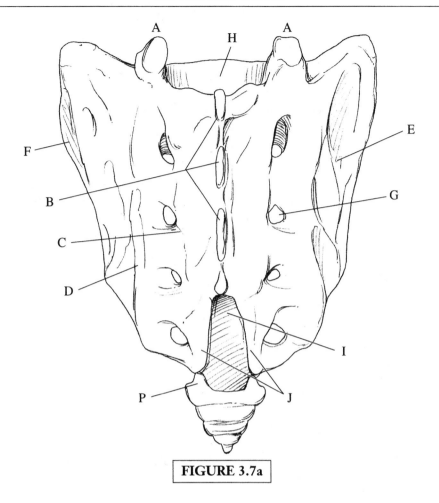

FIGURE 3.7a

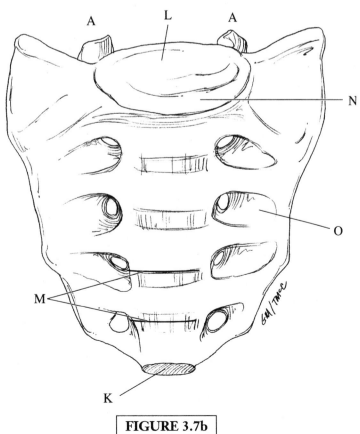

FIGURE 3.7b

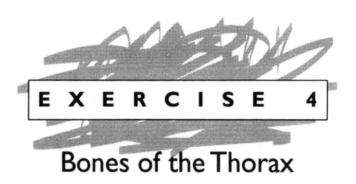

EXERCISE 4

Bones of the Thorax

The 'thoracic cage' is composed of the sternum and twelve pairs of ribs enwrapping the area from the vertebral column posteriorly to the sternum anteriorly. These skeletal structures play a role in four bodily functions: ventilation and exhalation (respiration), protection of thoracic contents, regulation of intrathoracic and intra-abdominal pressure, and movement of the upper limb.

STERNUM

The sternum (FIGURE 4.1) is described in three parts: the manubrium, body, and xiphoid process. The *manubrium* (A) is the most superior portion of the sternum. The superior surface shows the *jugular notch* (B), on either side of which is an *articular surface* (C) for the corresponding clavicle. Just inferior to the sternoclavicular joint an articular surface for the first rib is found. Color the manubrium yellow.

The *body* (D) (color orange) is the largest part of the sternum and articulates with the third through seventh costal cartilages (label these accordingly in blue pencil). An important landmark on the sternum is the *Angle of Lewis* (E), a usually prominent ridge at the junction of the manubrium and body. This ridge is palpable (capable of being felt) and is important because it indicates the level of articulation of the costal cartilage of the second rib to the sternum. Try to palpate it on yourself!

The most inferior portion of the sternum is the *xiphoid process* (F). This process may be bifid (cleft in two). It articulates partially with the costal cartilage of the seventh rib. Color the xiphoid process red.

RIBS

The bony thorax includes 12 pair of ribs; sometimes differentiated as 'true' or 'false' ribs. This description is a misnomer, all twelve are truly ribs! In anatomical fact, however, only the first seven pair of ribs articulate directly with both the vertebral column posteriorly and, via a costal cartilage, with the sternum anteriorly. Ribs 8-10 articulate with the vertebral column posteriorly but articulate anteriorly by joining the costal cartilage of the rib above. Ribs 11 and 12 remain free anteriorly. On FIGURE 4.1 designate these ribs with pencil lines as follows: ribs 1-7 green; ribs 8-10 sky blue; ribs 11-12 blue.

Another descriptive method is that of 'typical' and 'atypical' ribs. The components of a typical rib are shown in FIGURE 4.2. Each typical rib has a vertebral and sternal extremity with an intervening body. Find the following portions of a typical rib in this figure: *head* (A), with an articular surface divided into two *demifacets* by a small ridge. The rib articulates with both the body of its own vertebra, and with the body of the vertebra above, via these demi facets.

The *neck* (B) of the rib is about one inch in length and is located just lateral to the head. A *tubercle* (C) is found at the junction of the neck and body of the rib. The tubercle also shows a facet for articulation with the transverse process of its own vertebra. The *angle* (D) of the rib is an oblique ridge on the external surface, lateral to the tubercle, where an obvious change in the curvature occurs. Typical ribs also show a *costal groove* (E) on the internal surface, along and just superior to the inferior border.

Atypical ribs include the first, second, eleventh, and twelfth (FIGURE 4.3). The *first rib* (F) is the shortest and has the greatest curvature. It is flattened in a transverse plane, presenting superior and inferior surfaces. Distinguishing characteristics of the first rib include:

Head showing no division of the articular facet (1)
Neck (2)
Thick and prominent tubercle (3)
Absence of an angle
Two shallow grooves on the superior surface for the subclavian artery (4) and vein (5), with an intervening tubercle for the attachment of the anterior scalene muscle (6).
Lack of a costal groove

The *second rib* (G) is a transition form between the first rib and a typical rib. It has a curvature similar to the first rib but it is not quite as flattened; the angle is slight and close to the tubercle.

The *eleventh* (I) and *twelfth* (J) *ribs* share two structural similarities: a single articular facet on the head, and a lack of either a neck or tubercle. The eleventh rib has a very shallow costal groove, and the twelfth has none.

❓ FOR REVIEW AND THOUGHT

Describe the course and articular attachments of a typical rib.

Would individual ribs play different roles in inspiration and expiration?

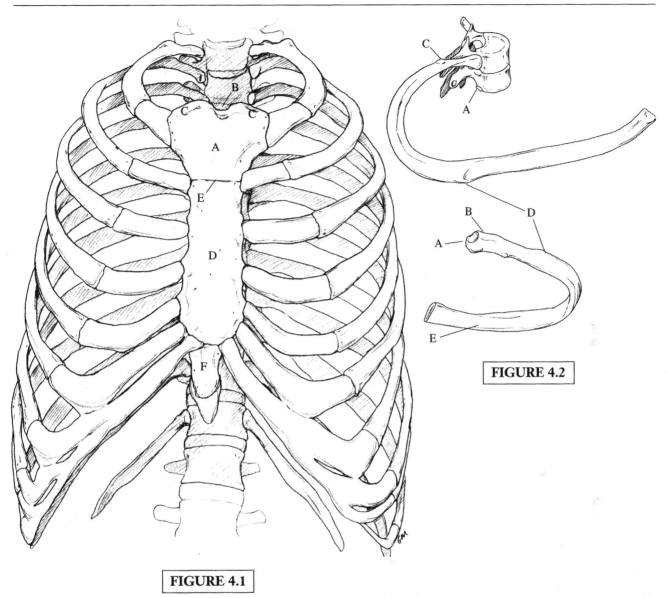

FIGURE 4.1

FIGURE 4.2

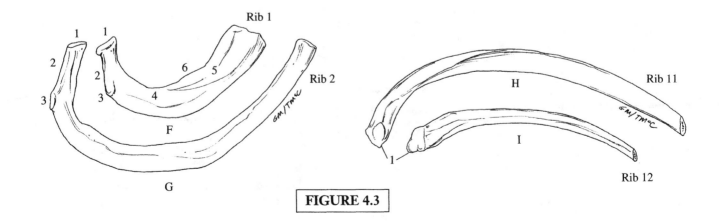

FIGURE 4.3

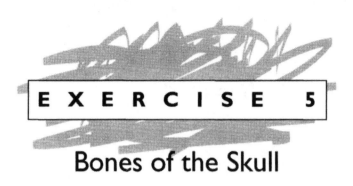

EXERCISE 5

Bones of the Skull

We will finish our learning of the skeletal system with study of the bony skull. For instructional purposes we will separate the skull into facial and cranial portions. This division is only somewhat arbitrary because some functional differences do exist between these portions. The bones of the face are involved in respiration, ventilation, mastication, and speech: not to mention their role in defining our 'look'. The cranial bones function in protection of the brain, cranial nerves, and intracranial vasculature.

Each of the bones of the face are shown individually on the facing page (FIGURE 5.1) and each has a color bar beneath it. Fill in this bar with the color designated and use the same color in the complete skull views thereafter.

THE FACE

Eight named bones participate in facial structure. Six of these are paired, producing a total of fourteen. Of the facial bones the *mandible* (color bar: green) is perhaps the most striking, and one might say, the most independent. The mandible develops in separate halves which unite in a midline suture: the symphysis menti. Three major structural components are described: the *body* (A), *ramus* (B), and *angle* (C). Find these on yourself by placing your index fingers on each angle. Slide your fingers anteriorly along each body until they meet at the mentum (L. 'chin'). Now retrace your path back to the angle and slide your fingers toward your ears along the ramus. The ramus terminates by diverging into the *coronoid* (D) and *condyloid* (E) *processes*. The coronoid process serves as a site of muscle attachment while the condyloid process articulates with the mandibular fossa of the temporal bone to form the temporomandibular joint. Between these two processes is the *mandibular notch* (F). On the inner side of each body find the *mandibular foramen* (G), through which the inferior alveolar branch of the mandibular nerve enters the jaw to provide sensory innervation to the teeth and gums. (It is here that the dentist anesthesizes the lower jaw.) The bodies of the mandible are also enhanced by the *alveolar processes* (H), which hold the teeth. Find the *genoid tubercle* (I) (G., geneion; the chin; L., genu; bent) on the inner surface

of the junction of the two bodies. This serves as a site of muscle attachment. Finally, find the *mental foramina* (J) on the anterior surface of each half of the mandible. The mental nerve, a small sensory branch of the inferior alveolar nerve, exits this opening to reach the chin.

The upper jaw is composed of the two *maxillae* (color bar: yellow) which join at the intermaxillary suture. Each maxilla is complex in form and includes a significant portion of the face as well as the inferomedial portion of the floor of the orbit (*orbital surface*, K). The two join anteriorly at the intermaxillary suture. Superficially the maxillae present a *body* (L); with *facial* (M) and *infratemporal* (N) *surfaces*, and *frontal* (O) and *zygomatic processes* (P). The body of the maxilla is a hollowed sinus lined with mucus membrane continuous with that of the nasal mucosa. (A situation you are familiar with if you suffer from hayfever or other sinus problems.) Horizontal extensions of the maxilla medially (*palatine processes*, Q) form the anterior two-thirds of the hard palate. Other significant features of the maxilla include the *alveolar process* (R), housing the upper teeth, and the *infraorbital foramen* (S) from which a portion of the maxillary nerve exits to supply sensory innervation to the skin of the cheek. Follow this opening into the floor of the orbit and find the *infraorbital sulcus* (T) *and canal* (U).

ⓘ FOR REVIEW AND THOUGHT

In our study of the lower limb we reviewed Wolff's Law, a concept stating that bone responds to levels of stress, or lack thereof, by adapting its structure. The edentulous (toothless) mandible is another example of this phenomenon. The removal of teeth from the mandible results in bone loss from the alveolar processes; leaving the mandible 'bar like'.

What consequences might accrue from such a condition?

What procedure is common in dentistry today to avert such possible consequences?

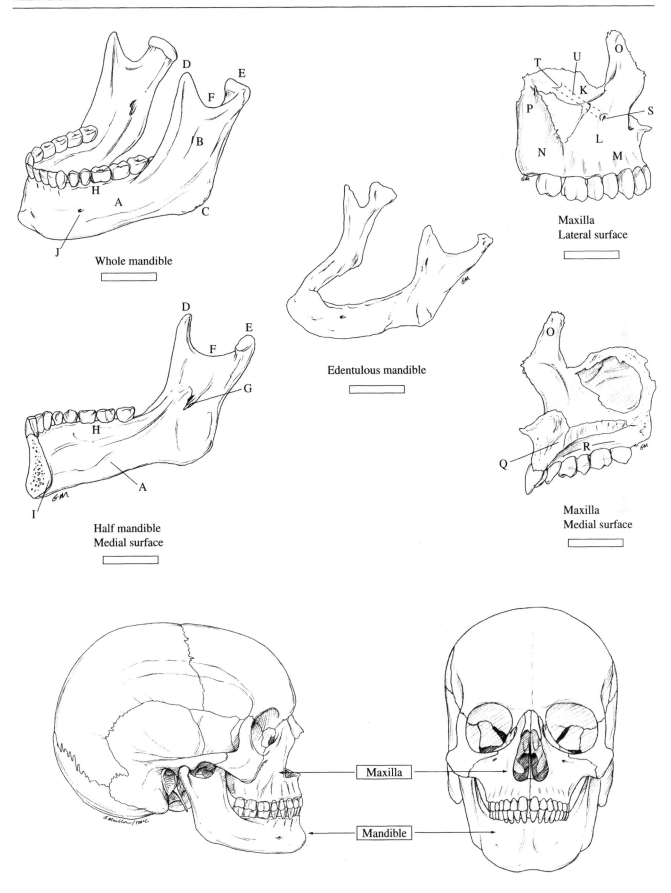

Whole mandible

Half mandible
Medial surface

Edentulous mandible

Maxilla
Lateral surface

Maxilla
Medial surface

Maxilla

Mandible

FIGURE 5.1

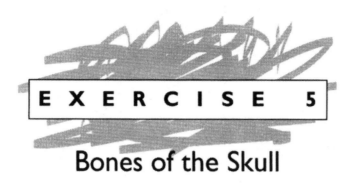

EXERCISE 5

Bones of the Skull

THE FACE

Two small *nasal bones* (color bar: purple)(FIGURE 5.2) border the superomedial aspect of the frontal processes of the maxillae and the frontal bone. This is the extent of the external skeleton of the nose. You can get an appreciation of just how small these two bones are by placing an index finger at the superomedial corner of each eye and sliding them inferiorly until you reach cartilage (perhaps one inch).

The two *zygomatic bones* (color bar: red) are perhaps the most interesting in terms of their impact on facial features. These 'cheekbones' present a *lateral surface* (A) and *frontal* (B) and *temporal* (C) processes. Each also forms a large portion of the lateral wall of the orbit (D).

Paired *lacrimal* (color bar: blue) bones are found at the anteromedial corner of each orbit. Each shows a *sulcus* (E); a grooved entrance into the nasolacrimal duct.

The *palatine* bones (color bar: orange) form the posterior extensions of the upper jaw. Each has a *perpendicular plate* (F) forming a part of the medial wall of the maxillary sinus and a *horizontal plate* (G) forming the posterior one-third of the hard palate.

The *inferior nasal conchae* (color bar: brown) articulate with the medial walls of the maxillae via a *maxillary process* (H). The conchae hang into the nasal cavity in a scroll-like fashion and are covered with nasal mucosa; serving to increase the surface area of the nasal cavity.

The tiny, and quite fragile, *vomer* (color bar: green) forms a portion of the nasal septum. It articulates superiorly with the palatine and sphenoid bones.

Note: in some anatomy texts the inferior nasal conchae and vomer are listed among the bones of the cranium.

❓ FOR REVIEW AND THOUGHT

Processes of what two bones form the hard palate?

On the facial bones find the supra and infraorbital foramina (the supraorbital is often a notch rather than a foramen). Notice that these fall in a perpendicular line with the mental foramen on the mandible. This will be of importance during our study of the cranial nerves because a branch of each division of the trigeminal nerve exits from each of these foramina to reach the face.

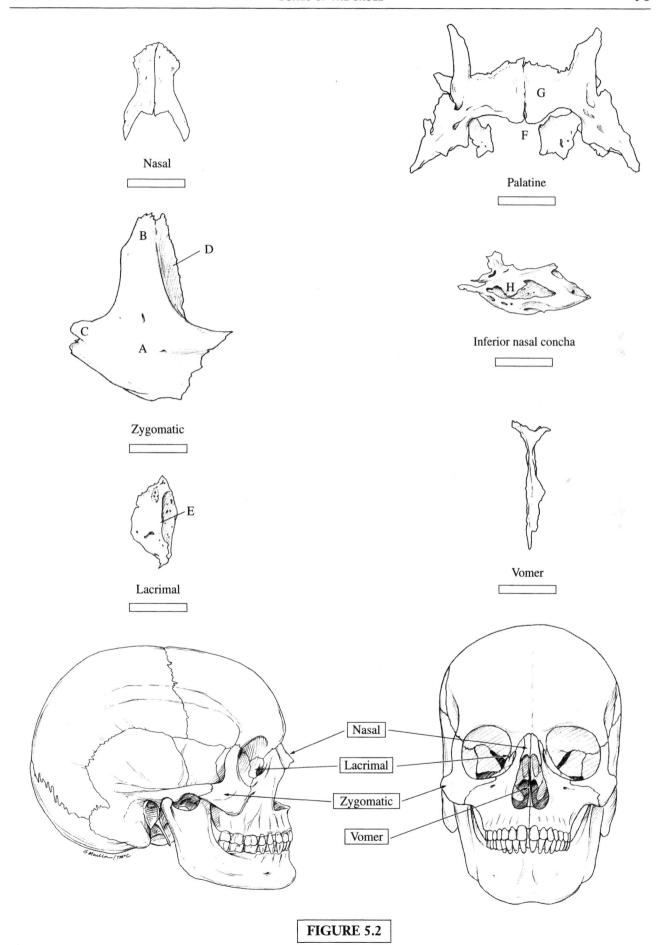

Nasal

Palatine

Zygomatic

Inferior nasal concha

Lacrimal

Vomer

FIGURE 5.2

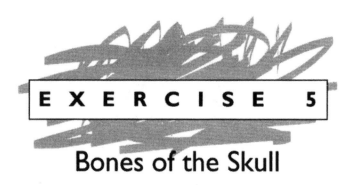

E X E R C I S E   5

Bones of the Skull

THE CRANIUM

Six bones are involved in the formation of the cranium. Two of these are paired, producing a total of eight. All are shown in the four views of the skull in FIGURE 5.3. Let's begin our learning with discussion of the *frontal* bone: the 'forehead', literally the front of the head (color bar: blue-green). This large bone extends posteriorly to nearly the apex of the cranium where it articulates with both *parietal* bones. This large sweeping and smooth area is described as the squamous (platelike) portion. The frontal bone presents orbital portions forming nearly the entire vault (roof) of each orbit as well as *zygomatic processes* (A), and *nasal* (B), and *supraorbital margins* (C). The frontal bones also contains sinuses lined with nasal mucosa (again, an all too frequent source of discomfort to those with 'sinus problems'). On the internal surface find the *frontal crest* (D).

The paired parietal bones (color bar: red-orange) form the posterior half of the lateral and superior portions of the cranium. They articulate with one another medially along the sagittal suture, and with the *frontal bone* anteriolly, the *temporal* and *sphenoid* bones laterally, and the *occipital bone* posteriorly. The external surface shows *superior* (E) and *inferior temporal lines* (F). Internally find the *groove for the transverse and sigmoid (S-shaped) sinuses* (G).

The paired *temporal* bones (color bar: purple) are described as having squamous (flat), petrous (rock-like), and tympanic (bell-like, or resonant) portions. The squamous portion is external and shows a *zygomatic process* (H), which combines with the temporal process of the zygomatic bone to form the zygomatic arch. On the inferior surface of the zygomatic process find the mandibular fossa (I) for articulation with the condyloid process of the

mandible. The petrous portion is more complex, housing the internal ear and several important branches of cranial nerves. Significant external features include the *mastoid* (J) and *styloid processes* (K), with the intervening *stylomastoid foramen* (L). Internally find the *groove for the sigmoid sinus* (G), the *carotid canal* (M), and the *internal acoustic meatus* (N). The tympanic portion shows the *external acoustic meatus* (O).

The occipital bone (color bar: yellow) forms the posteroinferior wall of the cranium. The most obvious feature of this bone is the large *occipital foramen* (P), also called the *foramen magnum*, through which the medulla oblongata passes. On each side of the external surface find the *occipital condyles* (Q) for articulation with the superior articular facets of the first cervical vertebra. Externally this bone also shows *superior* (R) and *inferior nuchal lines* (S), sites of attachment of important muscles of the neck. The *external occipital protuberance* (T) is a palpable landmark on the posterior surface of this bone. Find this on yourself now! Another feature of note are the paired *hypoglossal canals* (U) the route through which the hypoglossal nerves leave the skull. These are found most easily on the external surface.

On the internal surfcae of the cranial floor find the *cruciform* (cross-like) *eminence* (V), a significant landmark for several important structures. This cross delineates four quadrant areas, within which the right and left occipital lobes of the cerebrum and the right and left lobes of the cerebellum are protected. At the center of this cross is the *internal occipital protuberance* (W). Find grooves for the *transverse sinuses* (X) and *superior sagittal sinus* (Y) gathering here. The *basilar portion* (Z) of the occipital bone is found anterior to the foramen magnum and articulates with the sphenoid bone.

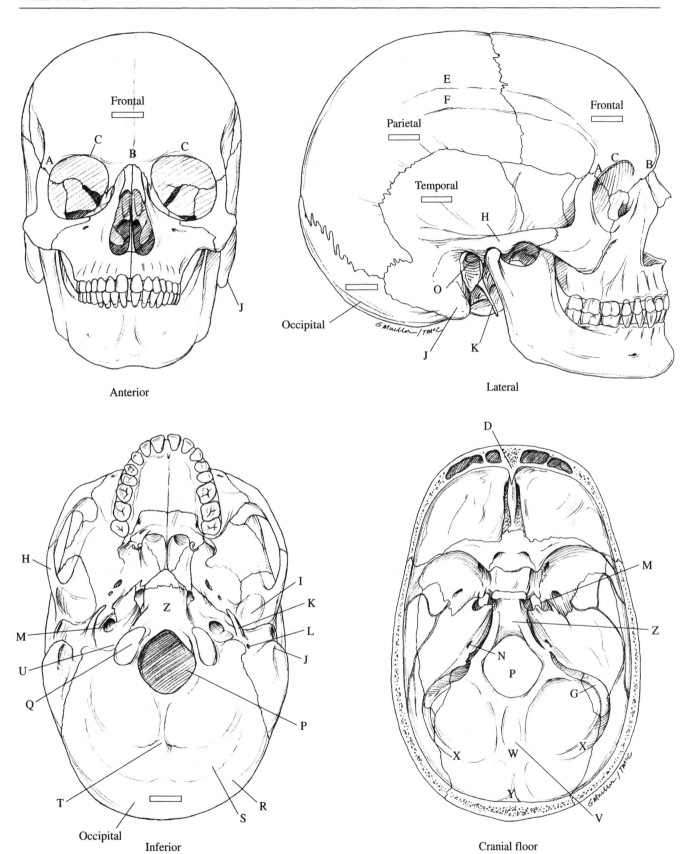

FIGURE 5.3

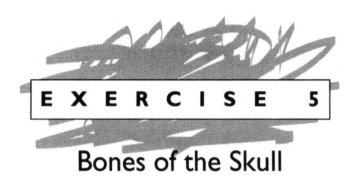

Bones of the Skull

THE CRANIUM

Two bones remain to be studied: the ethmoid and sphenoid (FIGURE 5.4). These bones are neighbors, centrally located at the core of the cranium, and structurally involved in a varied array of special purposes.

The *ethmoid* bone is fragile and complex, roughly cuboid in shape, riddled with sinus cavities, and found lodged between the media walls of the maxillae, anterior to the sphenoid, and inserted into the ethmoid notch of the frontal bone. *In lay terms behind the nose and between the eyes.*

Find the superior projecting *crista galli* (A) poking up between the roofs of the orbits. On each side of the crista galli are the *cribriform plates* (B) perforated for the passage of olfactory nerve fibers. Return to FIGURE 5.3 and find both of these between the orbital surfaces of the frontal bone.

The ethmoid also shows a *perpendicular plate* (C) which forms the superior portion of the nasal septum and *supreme* (D), *superior* (E), and *middle* (F) *nasal conchae*.

Combined with the previously studied inferior nasal conchae, these add significantly to the surface area of the nasal passage. All of the conchae are covered with mucus membrane. The ethmoid is also perforated with a *labyrinth of air cells* (G).

The *sphenoid bone*, is in our opinion, the key to understanding and visualizing the skull. It is a bone rife with foramina for passage of important nerves, veins, and arteries and its location is central within the skull. Several views of this bone are presented on the facing page.

Look at the posterior and anterior views! What do you see? A hawk, with wings spread and feet and talons hanging down to scoop up a prey? Or perhaps a bat? Whatever you saw record the image in your mind, it will aid you immeasureably in developing a three-dimensional understanding of this bone!

The central structure of this bone is the *body* (H) from which the *greater* (I) and *lesser* (J) *wings* spread. A key structure on the superior surface of the body is the *sella turcica* (Turkish saddle, K). The sella turcica is hollowed and contains extensions of the nasal mucosa. The slight depression on the supeior surface of the sella turcica is the *hypophyseal fossa* (L), occupied in life by the hypophysis (the rider in the saddle). Hanging from the junction of the greater wings with the body are *pterygoid processes*, each with *medial* (M) and *lateral plates* (N). Each medial plate is distinguished by a prominent hook at its inferior end: the *pterygoid hamulus* (O).

The greater wings present *temporal* (P) and *orbital* (Q) *surfaces*; the latter forming the posterior wall of the orbit. Each also has a tip projecting inferiorly and posteriorly: the *spine of the sphenoid* (R).

Because the sphenoid bone is centrally located within the structure of the skull many vessels and nerves enter or exit through this bone. Evidence of this is shown by grooves or holes. A prominent groove, the *carotid sulcus* (S) is found on each lateral surface of the body, formed by the passage of the internal carotid artery. Anterior and lateral to the body find the *foramen rotundum* (T), *foramen ovale* (U), and *foramen spinosum* (V). The former two carry cranial nerve branches out of the skull while the latter carries the middle meningeal artery into the skull. Tucked beneath the origin of the lesser wings from the body are paired *optic foramina* (W) through which the optic nerves pass to reach the retinae.

A final word about the body of the sphenoid. Like the maxillary, frontal, and ethmoid bones it also has a mucosal lined sinus as an extension of the nasal cavity.

JUST FOR FUN

Let us take you on a conceptual trip through the structures in and around the body of the sphenoid. Let your imagination come along! You are a pony express rider (hypophysis) sitting in the saddle (sella turcica) of a strong-hearted steed. Slung across the saddle and hanging on both sides are the mailbags (cavernous and intercavernous sinuses). As you 'hide' behind your horse's neck to increase speed your knees come to a nearly tuck position while your feet remain in the stirrups but push backwards (internal carotid arteries running alongside the saddle and bending sharply at the 'genu' to give off the ophthalmic artery to the eye).

Don't worry if this entire scenario doesn't make sense now. It should after you finish study of the cardiovascular and endocrine systems.

FOR REVIEW AND THOUGHT

What bones of the skull have sinuses?

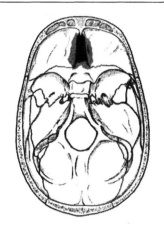

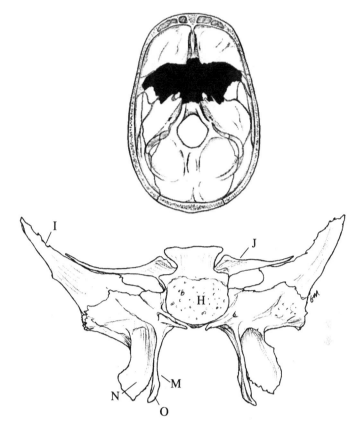

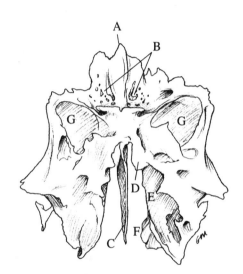

Ethmoid bone
Posterior surface

Sphenoid bone posterior

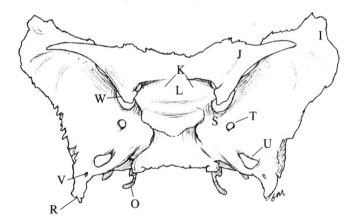

Sphenoid bone superior

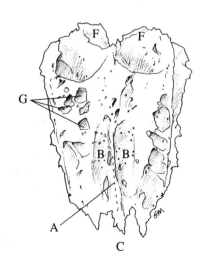

Ethmoid bone
Superior surface

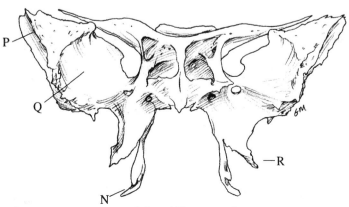

Sphenoid bone anterior

FIGURE 5.4

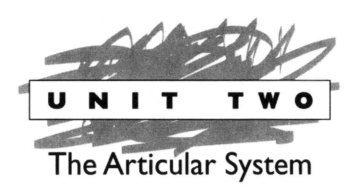

UNIT TWO

The Articular System

Joints are the functional sites where the skeletal and muscular systems interact (thus their positioning at this point in the text). The articulation of two or more bones is a joint. Generally speaking joints are constructed to allow or limit mobility. Those joints which favor mobility are more often injured than those which limit mobility. Thus: the glenohumeral (shoulder) joint is the most mobile and the most often injured. Use the scale below as a guide to joint structure and function.

mobility ⟵—————————————⟶ stability
often injured ⟵—————————————⟶ seldom injured
shoulder ⟵—————————————⟶ sutures of skull

Three main factors influence the stability/mobility equation of a joint: (1) the shape of the articular surfaces, (2) the strength of joint capsule and ligaments, and (3) the strength and orientation of muscles acting at the joint. In the treatment of joint injuries, or in the training to strengthen a joint, these factors must be kept in mind. For example: stability of the hip joint is due mainly to factor #1; that of the shoulder to factor #3; and that of the knee to both #2 and #3. The following categories of joints are usually described and are shown in FIGURE IIA-J.

NON-SYNOVIAL

Fibrous

Such joints are characterized by union via fibrous tissue. Three such types are described.

suture (G., to sew) – usually spanning a very small gap
ex: the sutures between skull bones (A)
syndesmosis (G. syndesmo-band; connective tissue) usually spanning a gap of some distance
ex: the interosseous membrane uniting the tibia and fibula (B)
gomphosis (G., nail, bolt)
ex: the teeth held in the sockets of the alveolar processes of the mandible and maxillae

Cartilaginous

Union is via cartilage, allowing limited movement. These joints are sometimes designated as primary and secondary. Primary cartilagenous are not considered true joints as they do not last throughout life. The epiphyseal plates of growing long bones are the best example of this. Two examples of secondary cartilaginous joints are:

symphysis (G., grown together) – intervertebral disks; pubic symphysis (C)
synchondrosis – costal cartilages linking ribs to the sternum (D)

Synovial

The greatest amount of movement is permitted in synovial joints. All synovial joints have several specific characteristics.

1. The articular surfaces of bones involved in a synovial joint are surrounded by a *joint capsule* of dense connective tissue.
2. The inner surface of this joint capsule is lined with *synovial membrane* which secretes *synovial fluid* into the joint.
3. Synovial fluid circulates within the joint and between the articular surfaces.
4. The articular surfaces are covered by a layer of *hyaline cartilage*.

gliding (plane) – nonaxial; very limited amount of movement; some gliding between surfaces
ex: intercarpal joints (E)
sellar (saddle) – biaxial; both articular surfaces are saddle-shaped (biconcave and biconvex)
ex: carpometacarpal joint of the thumb (F)
spheroidal; enarthrodial (ball and socket) – multiaxial
ex: coxofemoral (hip) (G)
trochoid (pivot) – uniaxial; permits rotation about a longitudinal axis
ex: atlantoaxial joint (H)

condyloid – biaxial; one articular surface is convex, the
    other concave (I)
    ex: radiocarpal joint (wrist)

ginglymus (hinge) – uniaxial; flexion and extension about a
    transverse axis
    ex: brachioulnar (J)

Synovial joints are often accompanied by, or associated with, bursae. These are sacs or cavities filled with viscid fluid and situated where friction between surfaces might develop. In some cases these sacs are in communication with the joint capsule. Three prominent examples are the subacromial, olecranon, and suprapatellar bursae.

Let's begin with study of the joints of the upper limb.

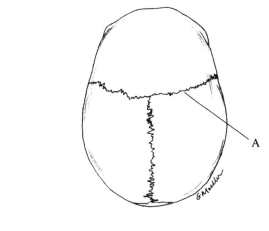

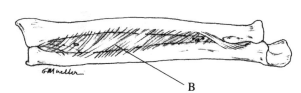

Fibrous

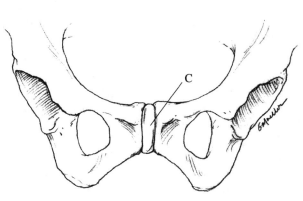

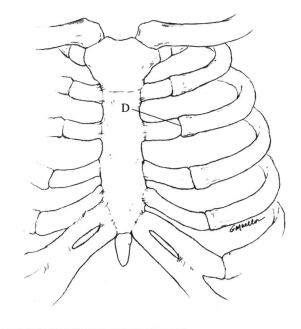

Cartilaginous

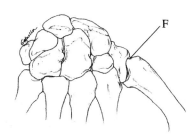

Synovial

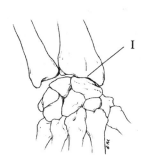

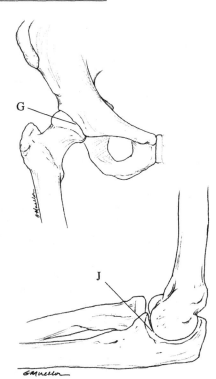

FIGURE II

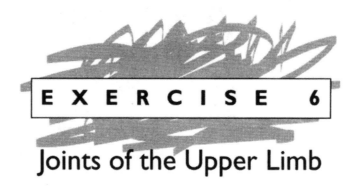

EXERCISE 6

Joints of the Upper Limb

STERNOCLAVICULAR

The union of the clavicle to the sternum (FIGURE 6.1) is via a plane synovial joint and therefore includes an *articular capsule* (A). A small *intraarticular disk* (B) intervenes between the bones and has attachments to the first rib and clavicle. An interclavicular ligament connects the two clavicles through the jugular notch.

ACROMIOCLAVICULAR

The acromioclavicular joint is also a plane synovial joint, and like the sternoclavicular joint has a *capsule* (C) and a small *intraarticular disk* (D). The *acromioclavicular ligament* (E) is associated with the integrity of this joint and is found on the superior surface of the joint capsule. Several other ligaments function in stabilizing the clavicle in relation with the scapula, these are: *coracoacromial* (F) and *coracoclavicular* (G) with *trapezoid* (G₁) and *conoid* (G₂) portions.

GLENOHUMERAL

The capsule of this joint surrounds the head of the humerus and attaches around the rim of the glenoid fossa: the *glenohumeral ligaments* (H). This capsule is somewhat thickened superiorly and extends to the coracoid process of the scapula as the *coracohumeral ligament* (I). Inferiorly the capsule is weak and counts upon several small muscles to aid in maintaining the stability of this joint. (The rotator cuff; to be described later in this text.)

This joint is multiaxial, allowing movement in all three planes of the body through all three axes of rotation: flexion/extension, abduction/adduction, and medial/lateral rotation (see pages 1 and 2 for a review). An additional movement capability at this joint is circumduction, a combination movement in which the extremity circumscribes a cone; brought about by sequencing flexion, abduction, extension, and adduction. Pitching a softball underhanded is a good example of such a sequence. Given the amount of movement allowed and the sparsity of structural attachment to the scapula is it any wonder the glenohumeral joint is so often subject to injury? Muscle strength is a key factor in the integrity of this joint.

HUMEROULNAR AND HUMERORADIAL

The trochlea of the ulna and trochlear notch of the humerus form one couple of this uniaxial joint; the other is the head of the radius and the capitulum of the humerus. In functional terms the humeroulnar joint is the main player allowing flexion/extension at the elbow. The radius tags along for the ride in these movements. One articular capsule encloses both joints. Also enclosed within this capsule is the proximal radioulnar joint. Here the head of the radius rotates in the radial notch of the ulna during the movements of pronation/supination.

The movements of pronation and supination are special to the forearm and hand. In the anatomical position the hands are supinated. Place your hands palms up on the table in front of you: this is supination! Now turn them over so the palms are on the table: this is pronation. Do this several times and notice that the movement involves the radius flopping forth (pronation) and back (supination) over the stationary ulna. The hand follows the lead of the radius. Why? Remember this: the hand goes with the radius! Students often confuse these movements so here is an easy way to remember them. To carry a bowl of soup, you have to supinate your forearm and hand. So picture this in your mind and think of *soup*ination [sic] and pronation!

RADIOULNAR JOINTS

The proximal radioulnar joint works in tandem with the distal radioulnar joint in pronation/supination. The articular capsule is thickened on the radial and ulnar sides as the *radial* (J) and *ulnar collateral ligaments* (K). The *annular ligament* (L) encircles the neck of the radius and attaches to the anterior and posterior edges of the radial notch of the ulna. It serves to hold the head of the radius in place during flexion/extension and pronation/supination.

The distal joint is a trochoid (pivot) joint between the head of the ulna and the ulnar notch of the radius. A small articular disk is found in this joint.

RADIOULNAR SYNDESMOSIS

The sturdy *interosseous membrane* (M) connects the ulna and radius throughout nearly their entire length. This is a fibrous joint.

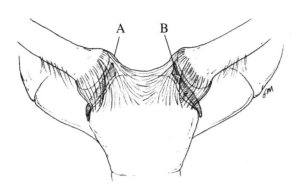

Sternoclavicular

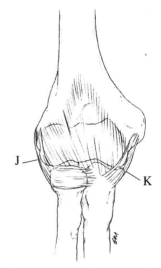

Humeroulnar & humeroradial

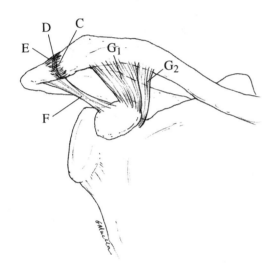

Acromioclavicular

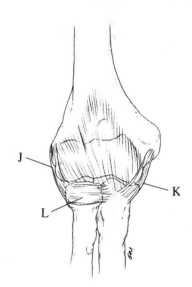

Proximal radioulnar

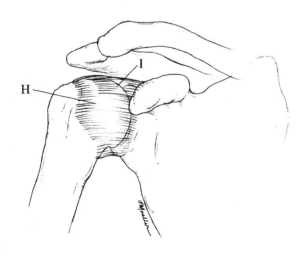

Glenohumeral

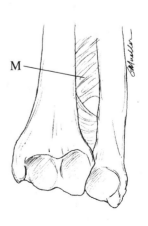

Distal radioulnar

FIGURE 6.1

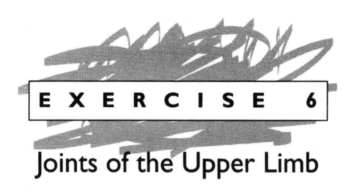

EXERCISE 6

Joints of the Upper Limb

RADIOCARPAL

The radiocarpal joint (A) (FIGURE 6.2) is, in fact, mainly a union between the expanded distal end of the radius and the scaphoid bone of the wrist. This is a condyloid joint allowing movement in two axes: flexion/extension and abduction/adduction; and therefore also circumduction.

INTERCARPAL

The plane joints between the carpals (B) allow only slight mobility between the bones in one row. A conceptual 'midcarpal' joint between the two rows may allow slightly more movement. At this time review the concept of the 'carpal tunnel' (p. 9) bounded by the tubercles of the scaphoid and trapezoid laterally and the hook of the hamate and pisiform medially. This tunnel is bridged by a layer of tough connective tissue: the flexor retinaculum. Use your yellow pencil to connect the pisiform and the hook of the hamate bone to the scaphoid and trapezium.

CARPOMETACARPAL

Very little movement is allowed at these joints for digits 2-5. This is not the case, however, for this joint of the first digit (thumb) (C) The carpometacarpal joint of the thumb is specially constructed to allow a great variety of movement. The basis for this is the unique capability in the structure of the saddle (sellar) joint. This joint involves two bones with reciprocating convex and concave surfaces. To aid in understanding this use the following mental imagery. Picture a saddle over the back of a horse. From one side of the horse to the other the saddle is convex. From the back of the saddle to the horn it is concave. Now imagine a rider in the saddle. Such rider may tend to slip off to either side or slide anteriorly and posteriorly. This is representative of the movements allowed at this joint; the most important being opposition, a combination of the above allowing the palmar surface of the thumb to meet the palmar surfaces of the other digits.

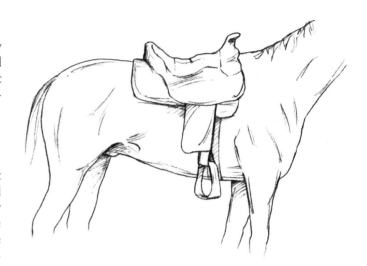

INTERMETACARPAL

The joints between the bases of the metacarpals are plane and allow very little movement (D).

METACARPOPHALANGEAL

These unions involve the heads of the metacarpals and the bases of the proximal phalanges (E). These are condyloid joints allowing flexion/extension and abduction/adduction, and therefore, also circumduction (although more limited than that of the glenohumeral or radiocarpal joints). The articular capsules of these joints are strengthened on the medial and lateral sides by collateral ligaments.

INTERPHALANGEAL

The joints of the phalanges (F) are uniaxial and allow only flexion and extension. Each joint, the proximal interphalangeal (PIP) and distal interphalangeal (DIP), is stabilized by collateral ligaments on both the medial and lateral sides.

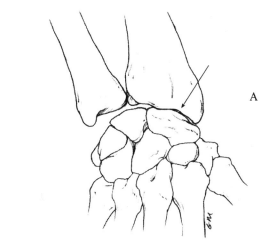

Radiocarpal

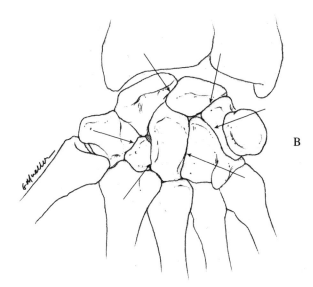

Intercarpal

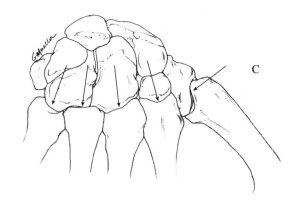

Carpometacarpal

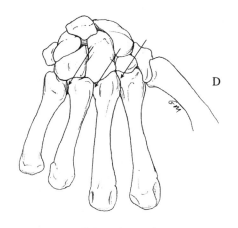

Intermetacarpal

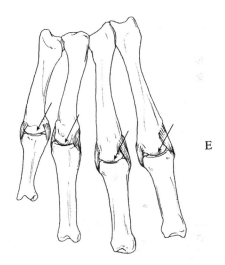

Metacarpophalangeal

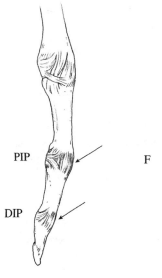

Interphalangeal

FIGURE 6.2

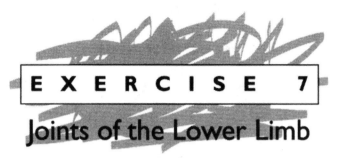

COXOFEMORAL

This joint possesses a strong articular capsule and a deep fit between the head of the femur and the acetabulum. Several thickenings of the capsule (FIGURE 7.1) are described as *ligaments*: *iliofemoral* (A), ischiofemoral (B), and *pubofemoral* (C). The proximal attachments of these ligaments are obvious. The iliofemoral ligament attaches distally along the intertrochanteric line and plays a large role in strengthening the anterior portion of the capsule. This is especially important in resisting the tendency for hyperextension at this joint (caused by the fact that the vertical line of gravity of the body falls behind the axis of the coxofemoral joint).

The ischiofemoral ligament supports the joint posteriorly and attaches distally on the anterior margin of the greater trochanter and intertrochanteric line. The pubofemoral ligament strengthens the medial portion of the capsule and attaches to the lesser trochanter. The *acetabular labrum* (D) is a fibrocartilaginous ring serving to deepen, and slightly enlarge, the articular surface.

An interesting feature of this joint is the *ligament of the femoral head* (E) passing from the acetabular notch to the head of the femur. This weak ligament carries blood vessels to and from the head of the femur. It is within the fibrous capsule of the joint as described above.

The joint is multiaxial, allowing movement in all three planes and about all three axes. Flexion/extension, abduction/adduction, and medial/lateral rotation, along with circumduction are the movements allowed. The depth of the acetabulum limits the amount of circumduction in comparison to the glenohumeral joint; due mainly to decreased abduction/adduction.

FEMOROPATELLAR AND TIBIOFEMORAL

The 'knee' is a compendium of ginglymus, trochoid, and plane joints. This surprising diversity of function is due to the unique structure of the joint (FIGURE 7.2); a structure remarkably weak in the articulation between bones and very dependent upon muscles, ligaments, and cartilage for stability.

The femoral condyles articulate with their respective tibial condyles with cartilagenous disks intervening (*medial* [F] *and lateral menisci [G]*). These structures are attached at their periphery to the tibia and to the joint capsule via *coronary ligaments* (H). The menisci serve to deepen the articulation, slightly, but act mainly as shock absorbers cushioning the force of biped activities. In a weight-bearing limb the femoral condyles roll and slide upon the tibial condyles in flexion and extension. Each meniscus is shaped to accommodate the appropriate femoral condyle. Notice the lateral meniscus is nearly circular in shape while the medial is 'C' shaped! As the joint reaches full extension the femoral condyles rotate upon the tibial condyles to put the joint into its most stable position. This is of great importance in a weight-bearing limb. During flexion and extension the patella glides along the 'patellar surface' of the femur.

At this point we must discuss a muscle

The popliteus muscle takes a tendonous proximal attachment off the lateral condyle of the femur and passes to an extensive muscular attachment on the posteromedial surface of the tibia. This muscle is a flexor at the knee, but more importantly functions to 'unlock' the femur from the stable position described above, allowing flexion to ensue. In the weight-bearing limb this involves lateral rotation of the femur upon the tibia, and in the free limb medial rotation of the tibia upon the femur.

The *patellar ligament* (I) envelopes the patella and serves as the continuation of the quadriceps tendon, attaching distally to the tibial tuberosity. The articular capsule of the knee joint is thickened by specialized ligaments. The *medial* (J) and *lateral patellar retinacula* (K) are seen on the anterior surface on either side of the patellar ligament. The *fibular* (L) and *tibial* (M) collateral *ligaments* pass from the lateral and medial condyles of the femur to the bone of their name. Notice the great difference in the structure of these two ligaments. The fibular collateral is short, cordlike, and separate from the joint capsule. In contrast the tibial collateral is longer, broader, flattened, and attached to the joint capsule.

Several important ligaments are also found within the knee joint. The *anterior* (N) and *posterior cruciate ligaments* (O) are the most obvious and the most *in*famous (certainly, at least, in the world of sport). They derive their name from the Latin crux (cross). The anterior cruciate passes from the anterior portion of the intercondylar eminence of the tibia to the posteromedial aspect of the lateral condyle of the femur. The posterior cruciate courses from the posterior side of the intercondylar eminence, and the posterior portion of the lateral meniscus to the anteromedial aspect of the medial condyle of the femur. These ligaments serve to limit and control movement between the tibia and the femur. **Each limits movement of the tibia in the direction of its name.**

Two small ligaments also bear mention. The *transverse ligament of the knee* (P) connects the medial and lateral menisci anteriorly, allowing them to move together during movements of the femur on the tibia. The *posterior meniscofemoral ligament* (Q) joins the lateral meniscus to the posterior cruciate ligament.

❓ FOR REVIEW AND THOUGHT

Study the collateral ligaments of the knee. Why is the medial more often injured than the lateral?

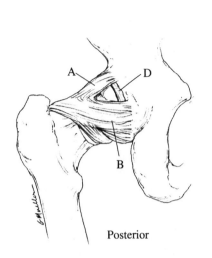

Posterior

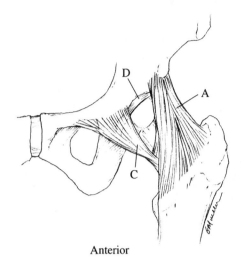

Anterior

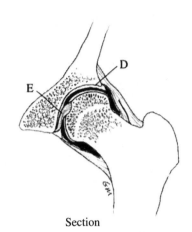

Section

FIGURE 7.1 Coxofemoral joint

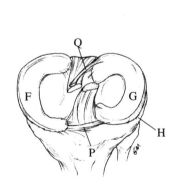

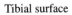

Tibial surface

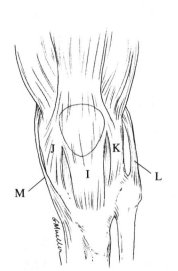

Superficial ligaments

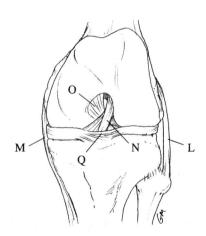

Anterior

FIGURE 7.2 Femoropatellar and tibiofemoral joints

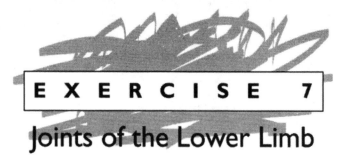

Joints of the Lower Limb

TIBIOFIBULAR

Proximally the head of the fibula articulates with the inferior edge of the lateral condyle of the tibia in a plane synovial joint. The distal union of these bones is of the fibrous type (FIGURE 7.3). *Anterior* (A) and *posterior tibiofibular ligaments* (B) bind the distal end of the fibula to the fibular notch of the tibia. A tough *tibiofibular syndesmosis (interosseous membrane)* (C) unites these bones for nearly their entire length.

TALOCRURAL

The 'ankle' joint is truly a union between the fibular and tibial malleoli and the talus. This is a hinge joint permitting movement in an anterior/posterior plane about a transverse axis. The unique mortise and pestle structure of the joint is enhanced by strong ligaments.

The *deltoid ligament* (D), a tough, wide, triangular-shaped, structure; provides support medially. This ligament has four commonly described portions, named according to their bony attachments: *tibionavicular* (D_1) (color yellow), *tibiocalcaneal* (D_2) (color orange), and *posterior* (D_3) (color red-orange), and *anterior tibiotalar* (D_4) (color red). Due to the strength of this ligament medial dislocations (sprains) of the ankle joint are not very common. In fact the ligament is so strong that forceful eversion (turning out) of the foot often involves a fracture of the medial malleolus.

Ligament strength on the lateral side of the ankle is much more suspect and inversion sprains of the ankle (the classic ankle sprain we have all experienced in which the plantar surface of the foot turns inward) involves tearing of these ligaments. Three lateral ligaments are of some importance: the *anterior talofibular* (E), *posterior talofibular* (F), and *calcaneofibular* (G). It is the anterior talofibular that most often suffers in ankle sprains! Color the anterior talofibular ligament green.

TALOCALCANEO (SUBTALAR)

This is a plane joint between the inferior surface of the body of the talus and the superior surface of the calcaneus.

It is surrounded by an articular capsule and strengthened by medial, lateral, and posterior talocalcaneal ligaments. This joint is involved in the movements of inversion and eversion.

TALOCALCANEONAVICULAR

This plane joint involves the head of the talus articulating with the posterior surface of the navicular bone, the sustentaculum tali, and the articular surface of the calcaneus. The interval between the navicular and the sustentaculum tali is spanned by the *plantar calcaneonavicular ('spring') ligament* (H). This forms a part of the articular socket for the head of the talus and also aids in support of the longitudinal arch of the foot.

CALCANEOCUBOID

The posterior surface of the cuboid and the anterior surface of the calcaneus articulate here in a plane joint. Two important ligaments are involved in the support of this joint: the *long plantar* (I) and *calcaneocuboid* (J).

The talocalcaneonavicular and calcaneocuboid joints are collectively referred to as the *transverse tarsal joint* (K). The name accrues from the nearly exact transverse line they form across the foot. This 'joint' is a conceptual one only; the talocalcaneonavicular and calcaneocuboid joints do not communicate anatomically. Functionally they act in inversion and eversion of the foot.

INTERTARSAL

These plane joints between the tarsals permit only slight movement.

TARSOMETATARSAL

These plane synovial joints permit only gliding or sliding movements. Three separate joints are described. The *medial* (L) involves the medial cuneiform and the first metatarsal and has a greater range of motion than the other two joints. (Compare this to the carpometacarpal joint of the thumb.) The *intermediate* (M) joint includes all three cuneiforms and the second and third metatarsals. It is the strongest of the three joints. The *lateral* (N) joint involves the cuboid and the fourth and fifth metatarsals.

INTERMETATARSAL

These are plane synovial joints allowing very little movement.

METATARSOPHALANGEAL

These are condyloid joints permitting flexion/extension, abduction/adduction, and circumduction. The first metatarsophalangeal joint is clearly the largest due to the size of the head of the first metatarsal. The range of motion allowed in these joints is less than that of the metacarpophalangeal joints of the hand. These joints are stabilized by collateral ligaments

INTERPHALANGEAL

These hinge joints permit flexion and extension and are strengthened by collateral ligaments. In most of us the lateral four toes maintain a partially flexed position.

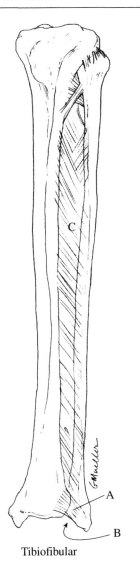

Tibiofibular

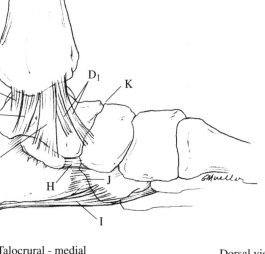

Talocrural - medial

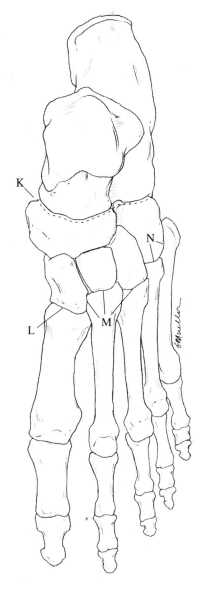

Dorsal view of foot

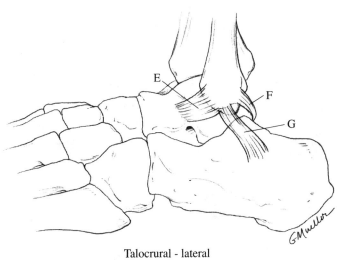

Talocrural - lateral

FIGURE 7.3

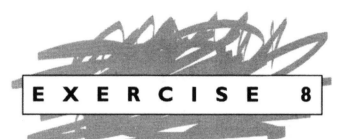

Joints of the Vertebral Column, Thorax, and Pelvis

VERTEBRAL COLUMN

From the second cervical through the first sacral levels of the vertebral column consecutive vertebrae articulate via three joints. One of these, the intervertebral disc, is anterior and non-synovial, uniting successive vertebral bodies. (see page 18 for previous description). Each vertebra (FIGURE 8.1) is also equipped with paired *zygoapophyseal joints* (A). These are plane synovial joints uniting successive vertebrae. The orientation of these joints changes from cervical to lumbar regions of the column and these changes may play some small role in the quantity and direction of movement allowed in each region. These changes are not sharply delineated but are transitional from one region to another (see page 18).

The paired *atlantooccipital joints* between the skull and C_1 (atlas) are specially structured to support the skull. These are synovial joints with the superior facets of the atlas articulating with the occipital condyles and allowing some flexion and extension; shown as nodding of the head.

The joint between the atlas and axis *(atlantoaxial)* is more complex; featuring three components. These joints allow lateral rotation of the head as in indicating disagreement. Paired synovial joints are found laterally between the superior facets of the axis and the inferior facets of the atlas. In addition the *dens* of C_2 articulates anteriorly with the posterior surface of the anterior arch of the atlas in another synovial joint. This joint is strengthened anteriorly by paired *alar ligaments* (B) coursing from the dens to the lateral margins of the foramen magnum and posteriorly by a singular *transverse ligament* (C).

THORAX

Thoracic vertebrae are additionally equipped with synovial joints for articulation with ribs. These *costovertebral* articulations include the union of the head of a rib with the demifacets of two vertebrae. An important element of the joint capsule is the *radiate ligament* (D) passing from the anterior side of the head of the rib to the bodies of two adjacent vertebrae. The *costotransverse joint* between the tubercle of a rib and the transverse process of its vertebra is dependent upon the *costotransverse ligament* (E). These joints allow/limit the movement of the thoracic cage in inspiration and expiration.

Sternocostal joints are found anteriorly. Ribs 1-7 articulate with the sternum individually via such joints and ribs 8-10 combine in one joint. The first pair of ribs unite with the manubrium of the sternum in a synchondrosis. Costal cartilages 2-7 join the sternum at individual synovial joints, each of which is strengthened by sternocostal and radiate ligaments.

PELVIS

An absolutely essential joint for the human upright stance is that between the sacrum and the paired ilia. These *sacroiliac joints* are synovial and are strengthened by several ligaments. The articular surfaces of the sacrum fit tightly into those of the ilia. Two dorsal ligaments are usually described. Spanning the gap between the bones are the *interosseus sacroiliac ligaments* (F); the primary support for this joint. The fibers bind the iliac tuberosities and the ala of the sacrum. *Dorsal sacroiliac ligaments* (G) are found more superficially and span the gap from the posterior surface of the ilium to the tubercles of the sacrum. *Ventral sacroiliac ligaments* (H) complete the support on the pelvic surface of the joint. The *sacrotuberous* (I) *and sacrospinous* (J) *ligaments* act as somewhat weak accessories in support of this joint.

The symphysis pubis is a cartilagenous joint uniting the two pubic bones anteriorly. A fibrocartilagenous *interpubic disc* (K) unites the bones. The joint is strengthened somewhat by *superior* (L) and *inferior* (M) *arcuate pubic ligaments*.

❓ FOR REVIEW AND THOUGHT

What types of movements are allowed between adjacent vertebrae in the cervical, thoracic, and lumbar portions of the vertebral column?

Are there any situations or life events when it would be beneficial for the sacroiliac and interpubic joints to become somewhat moveable?

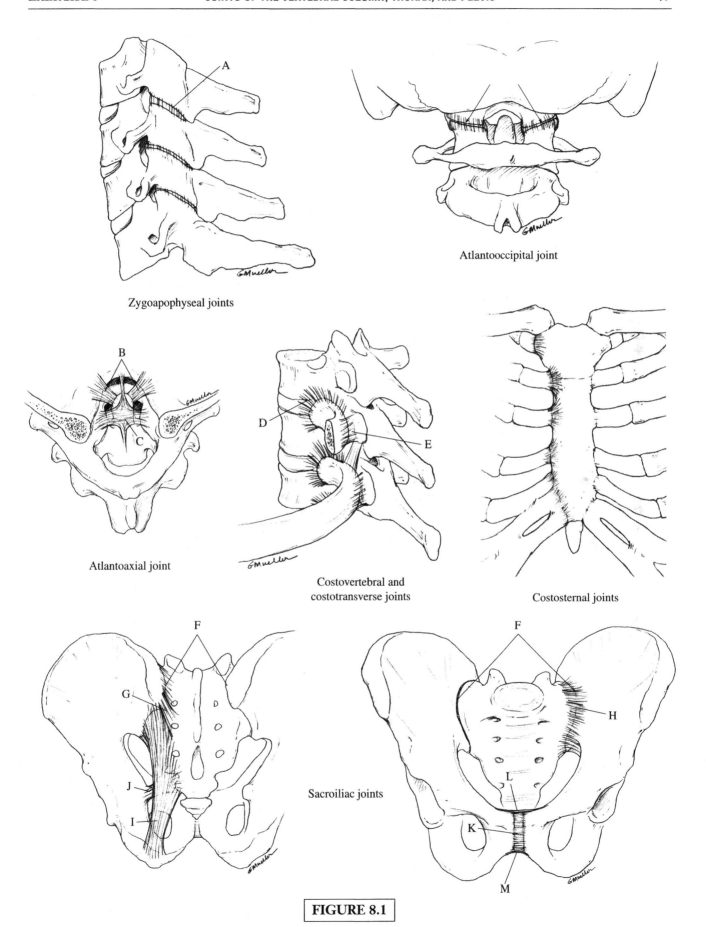

Zygoapophyseal joints

Atlantooccipital joint

Atlantoaxial joint

Costovertebral and
costotransverse joints

Costosternal joints

Sacroiliac joints

FIGURE 8.1

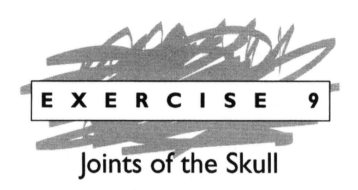

EXERCISE 9

Joints of the Skull

SUTURES

The facial and cranial bones (FIGURE 9.1) present a great many joints; most of them fibrous sutures that once spanned a large gap and now remain only as jagged lines. Use the various views of fetal and adult skulls to identify important sutures. One group of sutures are midline, separating the skull and face into equal halves. Find the following sutures on the surface: *mandibular* (A) (also called the mentis symphysis), *intermaxillary (B)*, *internasal (C)*, *frontal (metopic)* (D), *sagittal* (E), and the *median palatine* (F). In the cases of the mandibular and frontal only remnants of these sutures may remain. What did you notice about all of these sutures?

On the superior surface of the fetal cranium find the *anterior fontanelle* (G) at the junction of the *coronal* (H), frontal, and sagittal sutures; between the frontal and parietal bones. Follow the sagittal suture posteriorly to the *posterior fontanelle* (I) at the junction of the *lambdoid* (J) and sagittal sutures, between the parietal and occipital bones.

Other sutures define an individual bones contribution to various structures such as the hard palate, zygomatic arch, orbit, and nose. Find each of these and identify the bones involved.

hard palate –
zygomatic arch –
orbit –
nose –

GOMPHOSIS

A second type of fibrous joint found in the skull is the gomphosis, shown by the individual sockets in which the teeth are held in the alveolar processes of the mandible and maxillae.

SYNOVIAL

The skull also presents paired *temporomandibular joints* (K). As with all synovial joints this is enclosed by an articular capsule. The joint is formed by the condyloid process of the mandible fitting into the mandibular fossa of the temporal bone. A concave articular disk between the condyle and the fossa divides the joint into two chambers. A fibrous capsule and *lateral ligament* (L) passing from the zygomatic process of the temporal bone to the ramus of the mandible provide support. The joint allows some gliding as well as protraction and retraction of the mandible.

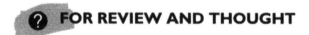

? FOR REVIEW AND THOUGHT

Why would the skull have only one synovial joint?

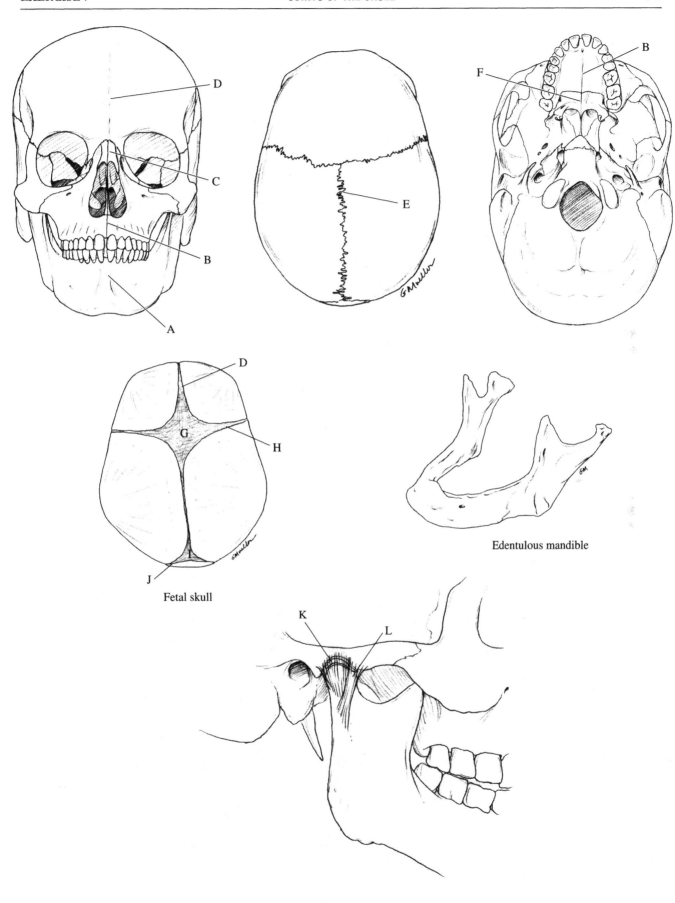

Fetal skull

Edentulous mandible

FIGURE 9.1

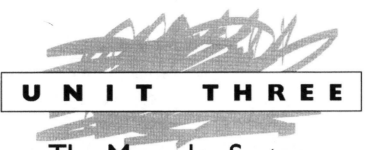

UNIT THREE

The Muscular System

Muscles are often described as having an origin and an insertion; with the origin defined as the more proximal, and more stable, attachment and the insertion the more distal, and more moveable attachment. This concept may become confusing when factors such as gravity and weight bearing are considered. For our purposes in this text muscle attachments will be described simply as proximal and distal.

The description of the muscular system here fits nicely because muscles cause movement of bones by crossing joints and contracting. Some of the muscles we will study cross only one joint, making their function very specific and clear. Other muscles cross two or more joints, adding to their functional capabilities but also diminishing their impact at any one joint. The functional union of muscle to bone is via tendons, a highly organized dense connective tissue of collagen fibers. Sometimes this union is very broad and flat and is called an *aponeurosis*.

TERMINOLOGY (FIGURE III)

Descriptions of muscles are based upon their architecture, attachments, appearance, and/or function.

ARCHITECTURE

fusiform – shows a fleshy belly in the middle with tendons at both ends; movement tends to be along the longitudinal axis of the muscle;
ex: biceps brachii

unipennate – the tendon is located along one side of the muscle and the fibers are obliquely arranged; yields a loss of movement but an increase in power;
ex: extensor digitorum longus

bipennate – the tendon passes longitudinally through the middle of the muscle with obliquely arranged fibers on each side;
ex: flexor digitorum longus

multipennate – muscle fibers radiate out from a central tendon;
ex: deltoid

triangular (or fan shaped) –
ex: adductor longus

ATTACHMENTS

coracobrachialis – proximal and distal attachments are on the coracoid process of the scapula and the shaft of the brachium (humerus)

brachioradialis – proximal and distal attachments are on the brachium and the radius

FUNCTION

extensor digitorum communis – the common extensor of the digits

flexor pollicis longus – the long flexor of the thumb

APPEARANCE

rhomboid major – a large muscle shaped like a rhombus

rhomboid minor – a smaller rhombus-shaped muscle

FUNCTION AND APPEARANCE

pronator teres – a pronator of the forearm and hand, long and rounded in appearance

pronator quadratus – a pronator of the forearm and hand, quadrate in shape

Prior to proceeding, return to the Introduction (page x) and review terminology, planes, and axes of motion.

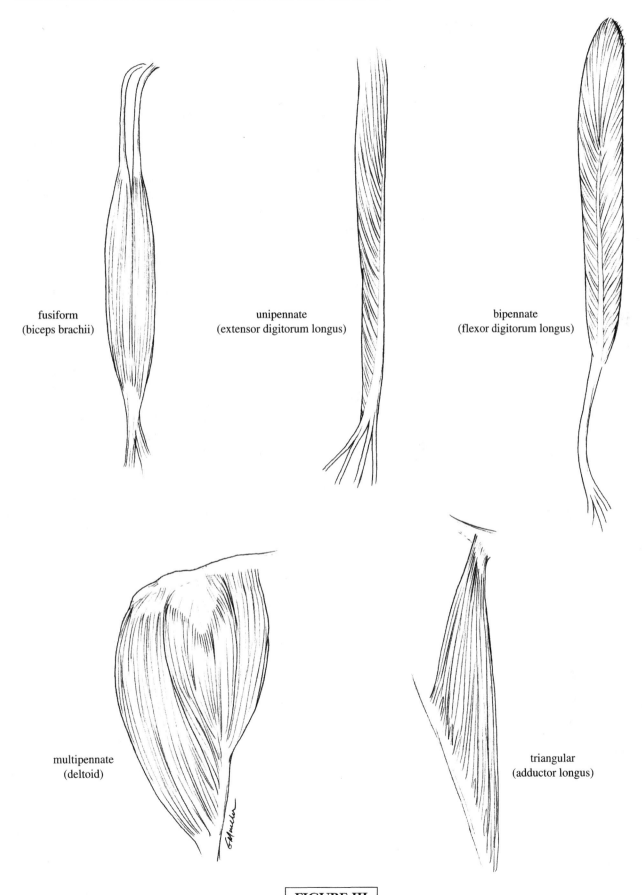

fusiform
(biceps brachii)

unipennate
(extensor digitorum longus)

bipennate
(flexor digitorum longus)

multipennate
(deltoid)

triangular
(adductor longus)

FIGURE III

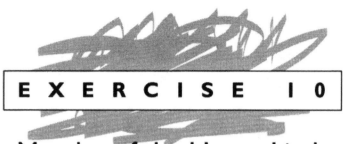

Muscles of the Upper Limb

THE PECTORAL GIRDLE

The muscles of the pectoral girdle serve to position the shoulder for a variety of activities and to anchor the girdle to the thorax.

ANTERIOR MUSCLES

The *pectoralis major* (A) (FIGURE 10.1) (color yellow) has an extensive proximal attachment from the medial half of the anterior surface of the clavicle (A_1), the sternum and costal cartilages of ribs 2-6 (A_2), and a weak portion from the most superior portion of the rectus sheath (A_3). The distal attachment on the lateral lip of the intertubercular groove is much more limited and the muscle fibers twist upon one another such that the abdominal portion attaches most superiorly and the clavicular portion most inferiorly, allowing a greater range of actions of the muscle. Given these attachments what movements might this muscle produce? Are these movements related to specific portions of the muscle?

Deep to the major lies the *pectoralis minor* (B) (color yellow-green). This muscle depresses the scapula. Its proximal attachment is from ribs 3-5, and distal to the coracoid process of the scapula. It also functions as a landmark for deeper lying structures in the axilla (armpit).

The *coracobrachialis* (C) (color green) takes proximal attachment from the coracoid process and attaches distally to the medial side of the humerus inferior to the medial lip of the intertubercular groove.

POSTERIOR MUSCLES

The *trapezius* (D) (color sky blue), like the pectoralis major, shows a large proximal attachment (from the skull to the spinous process of the twelfth thoracic vertebra) and a more limited distal attachment (on the lateral half of the spine of the scapula, acromion process of the scapula, and the lateral half of the clavicle). When the two trapezius muscles are viewed together they appear as a trapezoid: hence their name. Each trapezius is often described as having superior, middle, and inferior portions based upon the differing distal attachments and, in fact, these portions may act somewhat independently.

Deep to the trapezius are found several smaller muscles which aid in positioning the scapula. The *rhomboid*

major (E) (color blue) and *minor* (F) (color violet) both have proximal attachments on the spinous processes of vertebrae and distal attachments along the medial border of the scapula. The *levator scapulae* (G) (color brown) has proximal attachment on the transverse processes of cervical vertebrae 1-4 and distal attachment on the superior angle of the scapula.

The huge and powerful *latissimus dorsi* (H) (color light brown) presents yet another example of a muscle with an extensive proximal and small distal attachment. Proximally this muscle spans the distance from the sixth thoracic vertebra to the sacrum and iliac crest, and sometimes shows an additional portion from the inferior angle of the scapula. The distal attachment is on the intertubercular groove of the humerus.

The triangularly shaped *deltoid* (I) forms the rounded contour of the shoulder. *Clavicular* (I_1), *acromial* (I_2), and *scapular* (I_3) portions are usually described. All three combine to attach distally at the deltoid tuberosity of the humerus. Color these portions orange, red-orange, and red, respectively.

❓ FOR REVIEW AND THOUGHT

Given the attachments of these muscles what movements would they produce?

Pectoralis major (whole):
    clavicular portion:
    sternal portion:
    rectus sheath portion:
Pectoralis minor:
Coracobrachialis:
Trapezius (whole):
    superior portion:
    middle portion:
    inferior portion:
Rhomboid major:
Rhomboid minor:
Levator scapulae:
Latissimus dorsi:
Deltoid (whole):
    clavicular portion:
    acromial portion:
    scapular portion:

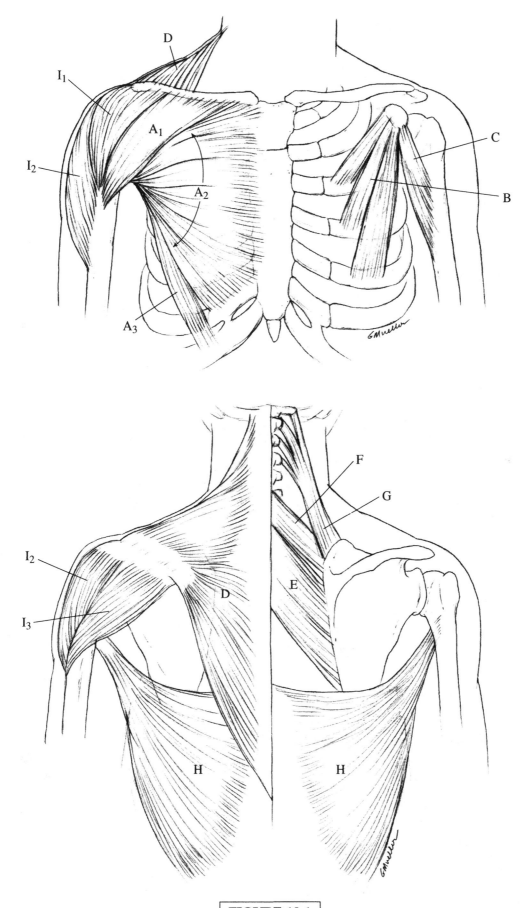

FIGURE 10.1

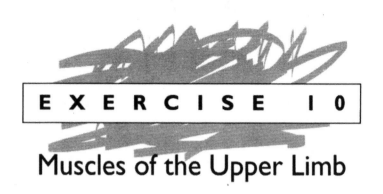

EXERCISE 10

Muscles of the Upper Limb

THE PECTORAL GIRDLE
POSTERIOR MUSCLES

Of the posterior muscles (FIGURE 10.2) four are involved in the 'rotator cuff'. This term is in part a misnomer: the four muscles do form a tight cuff on the superior and posterior surfaces of the head of the humerus, but only three produce rotation at the glenohumeral joint and another muscle which is a rotator is not a part of the cuff.

The *supraspinatus* (A) (color yellow) has a proximal attachment on the supraspinous fossa of the scapula and distal attachment on the superior tip of the greater tubercle. It functions in initiating abduction of the humerus. The first 10-15° of movement is due nearly entirely to this muscle after which the deltoid continues abduction to 90°, with the trapezius then assisting in further elevation (as in positioning the limb to throw a baseball).

The *infraspinatus* (B) (color orange) has a proximal attachment from the infraspinous fossa of the scapula and distal attachment to the greater tubercle of the humerus immediately inferior to that of the supraspinatus. It functions in lateral rotation of the humerus.

Attaching distally on the greater tubercle just inferior to the infraspinatus is another lateral rotator of the humerus, the *teres minor* (C) (color red-orange). Its proximal attachment is the axillary border of the scapula. It, too, is a lateral rotator.

The *subscapularis* (D) (color red) is the final member of this quartet, known as the 'rotator cuff'. Its proximal attachment is from the subscapular fossa on the anterior surface of the scapula. Distal attachment is on the lesser tubercle of the humerus (the only muscle with attachment on this tubercle).

As you have just learned three of these muscles have their distal attachment on the greater tubercle of the humerus, from superior to inferior. This can be remem-bered by the acronym **SIT**: **s**upraspinatus, **i**nfraspinatus, and **t**eres minor. To include the subscapularis simply add an s: **SITS!**

Understand that the *teres major* (E) (color yellow-green) is also a medial rotator of the humerus but is not involved in the rotator cuff. This muscle takes proximal attachment from the lateral border of the scapula near the inferior angle and passes to the anterior surface of the humerus to attach to the medial lip of the intertubercular groove. The tendon of this muscle is not involved in supporting the head of the humerus. The teres major is involved in medial rotation, adduction, and extension of the humerus.

The final muscle to be discussed is perhaps the most difficult to visualize and understand. The *serratus* (saw-toothed) *anterior* (F) (color green) takes proximal attachment via slips from the lateral surfaces of ribs 1-9 and distal attachment along the entire deep surface of the medial border of the scapula. The serratus anterior functions to hold the scapula to the thoracic wall, rotate the glenoid fossa upward, and act in pushing or punching activities.

❓ FOR REVIEW AND THOUGHT

You have now had an introduction to fourteen muscles functioning on the pectoral girdle. Each of these muscles has all, or part, of one of its attachments on the pectoral girdle. From this information decide which of these function primarily in positioning the girdle and which the humerus? Additionally, by studying the attachments, begin to develop a picture of what movements each of these muscles might produce, and conversely, what they might oppose. Work with a partner in a question/answer format and use examples from workday life, sports, dance, etc.

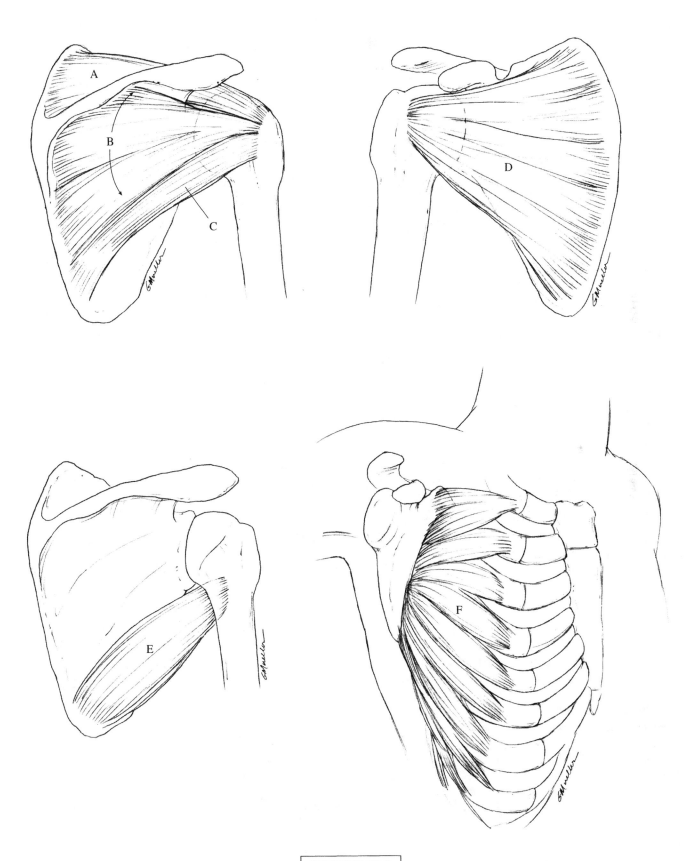

FIGURE 10.2

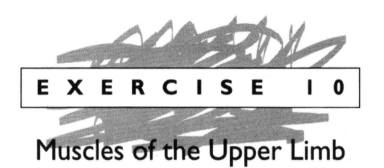

Muscles of the Upper Limb

ARM

The arm is the region between the shoulder and elbow and the muscles of the arm function at either, or both, of these joints. On the posterior surface of the arm is the *triceps brachii* (A) (FIGURE 10.3). As the name states it is a three-headed muscle of the arm. The three heads are *long* (A_1) (color yellow), *medial* (A_2) (color orange), and *lateral* (A_3) (color red-orange). Each has a separate proximal attachment and all three unite in a common distal attachment.

The *long head* is the only one functioning at both shoulder and elbow. It takes proximal attachment off the infraglenoid tubercle of the scapula. The *lateral* and *medial heads* take attachment from the posterolateral and posteromedial surfaces of the shaft of the humerus. The common insertion is into the olecranon process of the ulna. What movement does this muscle produce at the elbow joint?

Assisting the triceps brachii in extension is the small *anconeus* (B), with proximal attachment on the lateral epicondyle and distal attachment on the proximal ulna (just inferior to the olecranon process).

Two muscles occupy the anterior surface of the arm. The *biceps brachii* (C) is the more superficial. The *long head* (C_1) (color green) takes proximal attachment from the supraglenoid tubercle of the scapula and the *short head* (C_2) (color sky blue) from the coracoid process of the scapula. These heads unite near the midpoint of the arm and attach, via a strong tendon, to the radial tuberosity. This muscle also shows a dense aponeurotic band passing superficially to the medial side of the forearm. This structure, the bicipital aponeurosis, or 'false tendon of the biceps', is an important landmark in the cubital (anterior elbow) region. The biceps brachii is a two-joint muscle functioning in flexion at the shoulder and flexion and strong supination at the elbow (with this latter function enhanced during flexion).

Deep to the biceps brachii is the *brachialis* (D) (color blue). Its proximal attachment is from the anterior surface of the distal half of the shaft of the humerus. Its distal attachment is on the ulnar tuberosity. Unlike the biceps brachii it is a single joint muscle and functioning solely in flexion at the elbow and thus called the 'true flexor of the forearm'. It is the most powerful flexor at this joint.

❓ FOR REVIEW AND THOUGHT

Given the information you have just learned about the biceps brachii and brachialis muscles why are chin-ups easier to do with the palms facing you than facing away?

FOREARM, WRIST, AND HAND

Extrinsic muscles – those with proximal attachments on the arm or forearm and distal attachments on carpals, metacarpals, or phalanges.
Intrinsic muscles – those with both proximal and distal attachments on carpals, metacarpals, or phalanges.

Take a few minutes to review the bones and joints of the forearm and hand. Remember:

- the radius rotates about the long axis of the ulna during pronation and supination.
- the main articulation of the forearm to the wrist is that between the radius and scaphoid.
- the carpometacarpal joint of the thumb is a saddle joint between the trapezium and the first metacarpal.

FLEXOR ASPECT OF THE FOREARM

The muscles of the flexor forearm are nicely arranged in four layers. In general as you proceed from superficial to deep the muscles of each layer act more distally in the limb. This is not so for the deepest (fourth) layer.

Four muscles comprise the superficial layer. All have proximal attachment on the medial epicondyle of the humerus. They are: *pronator teres* (E) (color violet), *flexor carpi radialis* (F) (color light brown), *palmaris longus* (G) (color brown), *and flexor carpi ulnaris* (H) (color yellow). Using only the information you have right now what common function do all of these muscles have at the elbow?

The *pronator teres* attaches distally to the lateral surface of the mid-shaft of the radius.
The *flexor carpi radialis* attaches distally to the base of the second metacarpal.
The *palmaris longus* attaches distally to the fascia of the palm of the hand.
The *flexor carpi ulnaris* attaches distally to the pisiform bone.
Given this information what other function does each muscle have?

☽ JUST FOR FUN

Flex your right elbow 90°. Now place your left hand on this elbow such that the thumb is posterior and touching the lateral epicondyle of the humerus. Let fingers 2-5 lie anterior to the elbow on the skin of the forearm. In this position these four fingers represent the direction of the four tendons you have just studied: index (pronator teres), middle (flexor carpi radialis), ring (palmaris longus), and little (flexor carpi ulnaris).

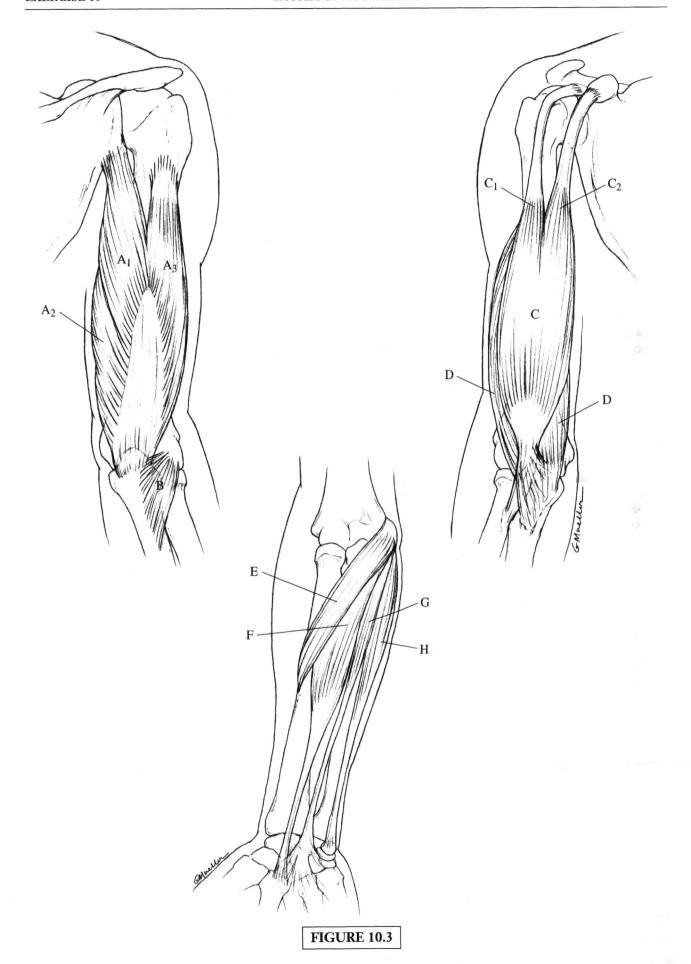

FIGURE 10.3

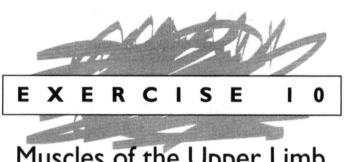

EXERCISE 10

Muscles of the Upper Limb

FLEXOR ASPECT OF THE FOREARM

The second layer of the flexor forearm houses only one muscle; the *flexor digitorum sublimis* (A) (FIGURE 10.4) (color red). (Many writers call this the flexor digitorum superficialis because in dissection it is seen before the muscles deep to it; but the reason for our preference for sublimis will be obvious shortly.) This muscle takes proximal attachment off the medial epicondyle of the humerus and attaches distally via separate tendons to the middle phalanx of digits 2-5. What joints do this muscle belly and its tendons cross? What movement is produced at each joint?

Two muscles occupy the third layer of the flexor forearm: the *flexor digitorum profundus* (B) (color green) and the *flexor pollicis longus* (C) (color blue). The flexor digitorum profundus takes its proximal attachment from the anterior surface of the proximal two-thirds of the ulna and the interosseous membrane. Four tendons pass from the belly of the muscle to the distal phalanx of digits 2-5, flexing the metacarpophalangeal joints (MP), the proximal interphalangeal joints (PIP), and most importantly the distal interphalangeal joints (DIP); while aiding in flexion at the wrist. This allows complete flexion of the hand for grasping: an action of profound importance; thus its name, and thus the use of *flexor digitorum sublimis* (its action is more sublime), described above. The *flexor pollicis longus* has a similar function in the thumb to that of the flexor digitorum profundus: flexion of the distal phalanx.

Return for a moment to page 9 for a review of the bones of the wrist and hand and the description of the carpal tunnel. The combined nine tendons of the sublimis, profundus, and pollicis longus are the travelers through this tunnel! They are accompanied by the median nerve. It is this nerve that suffers in carpal tunnel syndrome.

The fourth layer of the flexor forearm has only one occupant, the *pronator quadratus* (D) (color brown). This muscle has its proximal attachment on the distal quarter of the palmar surface of the ulna and distal attachment on the palmar surface of the distal quarter of the radius. Its only function is obvious and simple: pronation of the forearm (see page 40)!

❓ FOR REVIEW AND THOUGHT

Work with a partner and describe the attachments of the muscles you have learned. Using these attachments deduce each muscle's function(s).

How do the specifics of attachments impact the force exerted across a joint or joints?

List all the muscles you have studied so far that are flexors at the elbow joint.

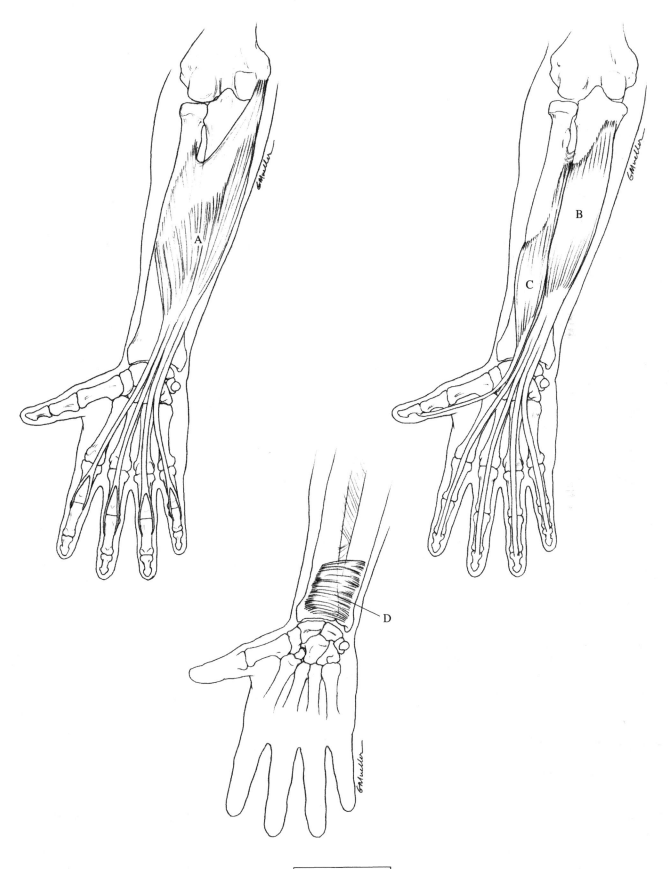

FIGURE 10.4

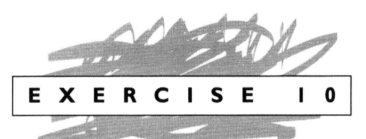

Muscles of the Upper Limb

EXTENSOR ASPECT OF THE FOREARM

The muscles of the posterior forearm are also arranged in layers (FIGURE 10.5). The superficial group all share a complete or partial proximal attachment off the lateral condyle of the humerus. As with the muscles of the anterior forearm those lying deeper have a more distal action on the limb. The *brachioradialis* (A) (color yellow) passes from the lateral supracondylar ridge of the humerus to the styloid process of the radius. It is a single-joint muscle producing flexion at the elbow: specifically flexion with the forearm in a neutral position (neither supinated nor pronated). How can a muscle described with the extensor compartment of the forearm be a flexor? Its proximal attachment is so high on the humerus that the muscle belly actually passes anterior to the axis of the elbow joint! In future work you will learn that the nerve to this muscle supplies the extensors of the arm and forearm.

The brachioradialis is significant in maintaining upper limb rhythm in sprinting. To examine this muscle on yourself place your right hand on the desk in front of you as if to pick up a glass of water. Now resist this movement by grabbing your wrist with your other hand. The muscle that 'pops up' is the *brachioradialis*!

The *extensor carpi radialis longus* (B) (color orange) and *brevis* (C) (color red-orange) have their proximal attachment off the lateral epicondyle of the humerus and distal attachments to the base of the 2nd and 3rd metacarpals respectively. Each acts in extension at the elbow and at the wrist. These two muscles are also significant in the making of a fist, which requires extension of the wrist in order to achieve maximum effectiveness. The *extensor carpi ulnaris* (D) (color red) takes proximal attachment from the lateral epicondyle of the humerus and the shaft of the ulna and passes distally to attach to the base of the 5th metacarpal. It functions in extension at the wrist with the longus and brevis, but more importantly in adduction of the wrist, in company with its counterpart on the anterior side (flexor carpi ulnaris). The extensor carpi radialis longus and brevis function similarly with the flexor carpi radialis to abduct the wrist! (Keep the anatomical position in mind.)

Extensor digitorum communis (E) (color yellow-green) passes from the lateral epicondyle of the humerus, splits into four tendons, and attaches distally via 'extensor expansions' on digits 2-5. This muscle extends and spreads the fingers and is a strong dorsiflexor at the wrist. Unique to this muscle are intertendinous connections, which provide the 'communal' function; but also limit independent extension of digits 3 and 4.

Extensor digiti minimi (F) (color green) is often a slip off the extensor digitorum communis. It attaches distally via an expansion on the fifth digit.

The *extensor indicis* (G) (color sky blue), sometimes also called *proprius*, has a proximal attachment off the posterior surface of the distal ulna and interosseous membrane and a distal attachment into the extensor expansion of the index (2nd) finger.

The deepest muscle of the posterior forearm is the *supinator* (H) (color blue). The name describes the function of this muscle. Proximally it attaches to the supinator crest of the ulna and the lateral epicondyle of the humerus. It wraps around the radius to attach between the radial tuberosity and the attachment of the pronator teres. It functions to supinate the forearm.

The second layer in the extensor forearm also includes the 'outcropping muscles'. These muscles form a bulge on the posterolateral surface of the inferior forearm. They have proximal attachment on the ulna, radius, and interosseous membrane and distal attachments, by means of prominent tendons, onto the thumb. Their tendons form the boundaries of an area at the base of the thumb called the 'anatomical snuff box'. Gentlemen of earlier eras put their snuff in this depression. Of more significance to the present discussion is the fact the radial artery passes along the floor of the snuffbox and the pulse can be felt by pressing the artery against the deeper lying trapezium and scaphoid.

The 'outcropping muscles' are the *extensor pollicis brevis* (I) (color violet) which passes into the hand to attach on the base of the proximal phalanx. The *abductor pollicis longus* (J) (color light brown) which, along with the brevis, forms the anterior boundary of the 'snuffbox', attaches to the base of the first metacarpal. The posterior boundary of the 'snuffbox' is the tendon of the *extensor pollicis longus* (K) (color brown) passing from its muscle belly on the ulna and interosseous membrane to the base of the distal phalanx of the thumb.

❓ FOR REVIEW AND THOUGHT

What muscles of the forearm act at more than one joint?

How do the flexor and extensor muscles of the wrist function in abduction and adduction of the wrist? Be specific in describing this!

You have studied four muscles with major functions in either pronation or supination: list these muscles! What do all of these muscles have in common regarding their distal attachment?

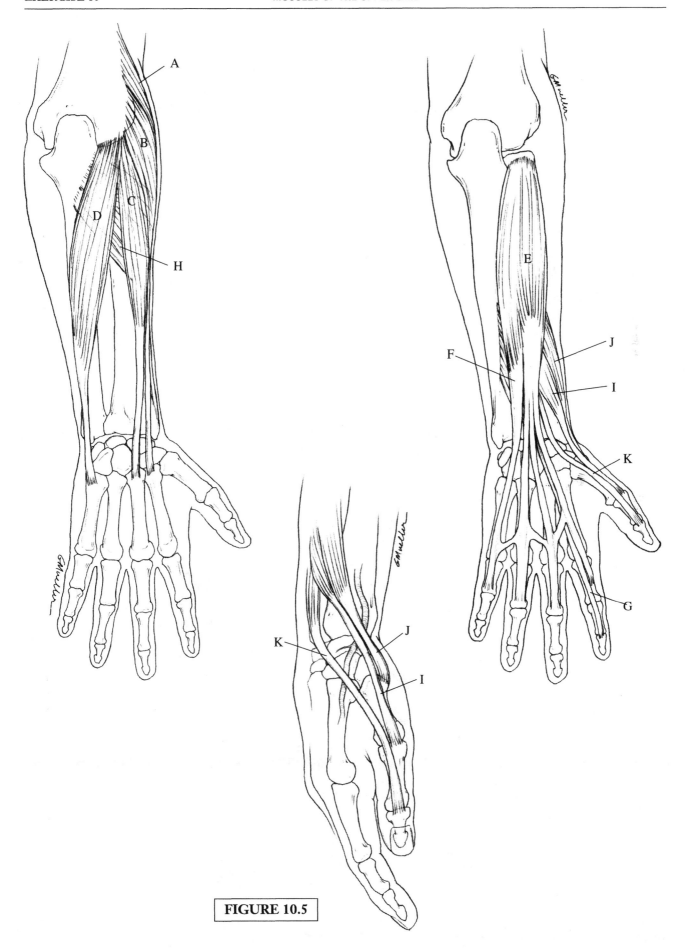

FIGURE 10.5

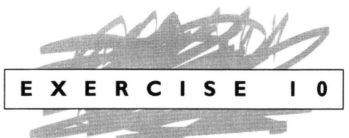

EXERCISE 10
Muscles of the Upper Limb

THE HAND

The muscles you have learned thus far are **extrinsic** muscles of the hand. **Intrinsic** muscles have both their proximal and distal attachments on the bones of the hand.

THENAR MUSCLES

Four intrinsic muscles function in positioning the thumb. Three of these are found in the thenar eminence, the raised pad at the base of the thumb. Notice that the palmar surface of the thumb is turned 90° to the other digits. Verify this by flexing digits 2-5 and then flexing the thumb. It moves across the anterior surface of these digits. The thumb is capable of an important additional movement: **opposition**. Opposition of the thumb brings the palmar surface in contact with the palmar surfaces of the other digits. What structural adaptation of the thumb which you have already learned allows this?

Of the thenar muscles (**FIGURE 10.6**) three are found in the thenar eminence: the *abductor pollicis brevis* (A) (color yellow), *flexor pollicis brevis* (B) (color orange), and *opponens pollicis* (C) (color red-orange). Of these the opponens is deepest. All of these muscles have their distal attachment on the proximal phalanx of the first metacarpal. The *adductor pollicis* (D) (color red) is found on the palmar side of the gap between the first and second metacarpals and has two heads: oblique and transverse. The functions of the individual thenar muscles are obvious by their names!

HYPOTHENAR MUSCLES

The hypothenar eminence houses the *abductor* (E) (color yellow-green), *flexor* (F) (color green), and *opponens digiti minimi* (G) (color sky blue). The arrangement of these muscles is the same as that on the thenar eminence but the amount of opposition is much more limited here.

LUMBRICALS

The four *lumbrical (wormlike) muscles* (H) (color blue) are unique in attachments and dramatic in function: capable of producing flexion and extension at different joints simultaneously. They take proximal attachment off the tendons of the flexor digitorum profundus in the hand, pass anterior to the axis of the metacarpophalangeal joints (MP) joints, and attach distally to the extensor expansions of digits 2-5. They produce flexion at the MP joints while maintaining extension at the interphalangeal (IP) joints. These small and simple muscles provide for a range of finger positions between complete extension and flexion. The next time you hold a hand of cards appreciate that these muscles are positioning your fingers to do so! **Especially if it is winning hand!**

INTEROSSEI

Seven *interossei* are present: *three palmar and four dorsal.* The *dorsal* (I) (color violet) pass from opposing sides of adjacent metacarpals and attach to the proximal phalanx of digits 2-4, while the *palmar* (J) (color brown) pass from metacarpals 2, 4, and 5 to attach to the proximal phalanges of the same digits. The dorsal interossei produce abduction and the palmar adduction. Note that the center point of these movements is the midline of digit 3. To remember the functions of the interossei use this acronym: **PAD**, palmar adduct and **DAB**, dorsal abduct.

❓ FOR REVIEW AND THOUGHT

Work with a partner in describing and understanding what muscles function in various positions of the wrist and hand! In order to do this use your hands in various situations and activities: hold a ball, grip a pen, strum a guitar, clap your hands, wave good-bye, hold a razor, button your shirt, brush your teeth, or fold your hands in prayer.

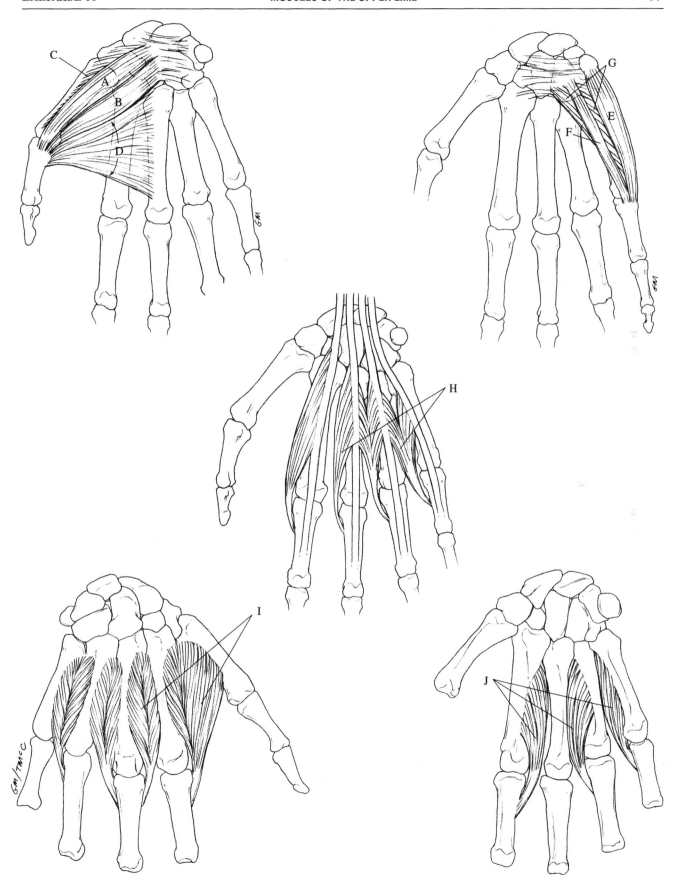

FIGURE 10.6

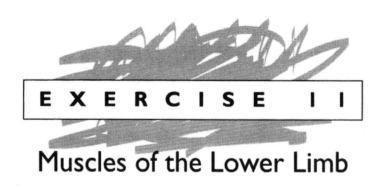

EXERCISE 11

Muscles of the Lower Limb

GLUTEAL MUSCLES

The gluteal region contains some powerful muscles used in locomotion and smaller muscles functioning in pelvic alignment and hip rotation. The most obvious muscle is the *gluteus maximus* (FIGURE 11.1) (A) (color yellow); a powerful extensor at the hip, functioning in such bold actions as running uphill, walking stairs, sprint starts, and getting up from a seated or squatting position. It takes proximal attachment superficially from the iliac crest, sacrum, and coccyx; and deeply from the sacrotuberous ligament. Distally it attaches to the iliotibial tract (a thickening of the fascia lata enwrapping the thigh) and the gluteal tuberosity of the femur.

Deep and anterior to the maximus are two more gluteal muscles; the *gluteus medius* (B) (color orange) and *minimus* (C) (color red-orange). The proximal attachment of the medius is between the anterior and posterior gluteal lines and that of the minimus between the anterior and inferior gluteal lines. Both muscles distally attach into the greater trochanter of the femur. They function in medial rotation of the femur, but more importantly in abduction of the femur.

The role of the gluteus medius and minimis in locomotion is critical. Contraction of these muscles in the weight-bearing limb overcomes the effect of gravity on the free limb, allowing this limb to swing through without dragging on the ground.

DEEP ROTATORS

Deep to the gluteal muscles are a group of small muscles all functioning in lateral rotation of the femur and referred to as the deep, or short, rotators. The *piriformis* (D) (color red) has a proximal attachment off the anterior surface of the sacrum and passes through the greater sciatic foramen to attach distally on the tip of the greater trochanter of the femur. The piriformis is an important landmark because the sciatic nerve usually exits the pelvis immediately inferior to this muscle.

As implied by its name the *obturator internus* (E) (color yellow-green) takes proximal attachment off the deep surface of the obturator membrane and the ischiopubic rami surrounding the obturator foramen. It exits through the lesser sciatic foramen to attach to the deep surface of the greater trochanter of the femur. The *superior gemellus* (F) (color green) and *inferior gemellus* (G) (color sky blue) are closely associated with the obturator internus in both attachments and function. The superior gemellus has proximal attachment on the ischial spine, the inferior on the ischial tuberosity, and both attach distally to the deep surface of the greater trochanter.

Two other muscles are found among this group of short rotators. The *obturator externus* (H) (color blue) takes proximal attachment from the rim of the bony margin of the obturator foramen and the superficial surface of the obturator membrane and distal attachment on the trochanteric fossa. Finally, the *quadratus femoris* (I) (color violet) passes from the ischial tuberosity to the intertrochanteric crest of the femur.

❓ FOR REVIEW AND THOUGHT

Compare and contrast the functions of the three gluteal muscles: maximus, medius, and minimus. Do this in terms of size, attachments, and role in various forms of locomotion. Relate these to activities of daily life.

Compare the 'short rotators' of the hip with the rotator cuff of the shoulder.

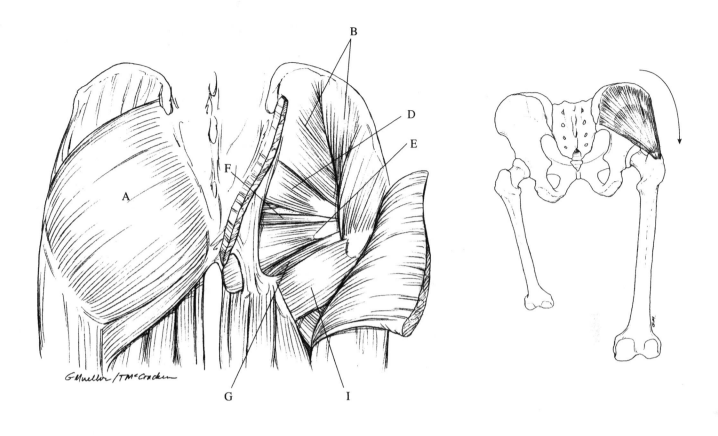

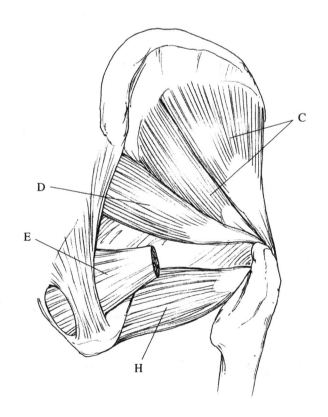

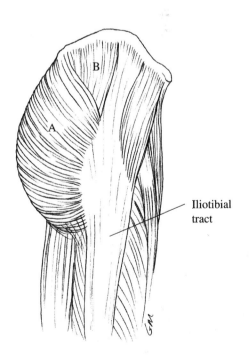

FIGURE 11.1

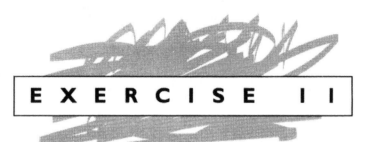

EXERCISE 11

Muscles of the Lower Limb

THIGH

The muscles of the thigh are descriptively (and generally functionally) divided into three compartments. This is accomplished by deep extensions of the fascia lata (deep fascia of the thigh) which attach to the linea aspera and define anterior, posterior, and medial muscle groups.

ANTERIOR THIGH

The predominant muscle in this portion of the thigh is the *quadriceps femoris* (A) (FIGURE 11.2). This four-headed muscle is, perhaps, the most important in the functional capacity of the human to locomote in a variety of ways: walk, jump, run, hop, and skip. It is the main occupant of the anterior thigh. One head, the *rectus femoris* (A$_1$) (color yellow), functions at both the hip (flexion) and knee (extension) joints. It takes proximal attachment off the anterior inferior iliac spine and attaches distally with the other three heads into the tibial tuberosity.

The remaining three heads take their proximal attachment off the femur. The *vastus intermedius* (A$_2$) (color orange) is the deepest of these and takes proximal attachment off the anterior shaft of the femur. The *vastus medialis* (A$_3$) (color red-orange) takes attachment from the medial lip of the linea aspera. The *vastus lateralis* (A$_4$) (color red) is the largest; taking proximal attachment from the lateral surface of the greater trochanter, the intertrochanteric line, gluteal tuberosity, and lateral lip of the linea aspera. Thus the vastus portion of the quadriceps femoris wraps nearly completely around the shaft of the femur! Distally this powerful muscle envelops the patella within its tendon of attachment into the tibial tuberosity.

The most superficial muscle of the anterior thigh is the *sartorius* (B) (color yellow-green). Its name derives from the Latin word for tailor, because of the tailor's habit of sitting cross-legged while working. The muscle takes a superolateral to inferomedial course from a proximal attachment on the anterior superior iliac spine to a distal attachment on the anterior aspect of the medial condyle of the tibia. In its course the sartorius passes anterior to the axis of rotation of the hip joint and posterior to the axis of rotation of the knee joint. Thus it functions in flexion at the hip, flexion at the knee, and lateral rotation at the hip: the very movements necessary to sit "Indian style" or to place one leg across the other thigh, as a tailor would work. Try this now yourself!

The sartorius also forms the lateral boundary of an area known as the femoral triangle, an important geographic landmark in the thigh. The medial border of this triangle is formed by the adductor longus muscle and the superior border by a tough fibrous band known as the inguinal (L., groin) ligament. The inguinal ligament runs from the anterior superior iliac spine to the pubic tubercle and is a geographic marker between the abdomen and the thigh. The femoral triangle contains several important vascular and neural structures. From lateral to medial these are: femoral nerve, femoral artery, femoral vein, and an empty space with lymphatic vessels and nodes. The mnemonic **NAVEL** will help you remember these structures from lateral to medial!

Two anterior thigh muscles form the floor of this triangle: iliopsoas and pectineus. The *iliopsoas* (C) (color green) is the more lateral. It is, in reality, a compound muscle formed by the union of the *iliacus* (C$_1$) and the *psoas major* (C$_2$). The psoas major has proximal attachment off the transverse processes, bodies, and intervertebral discs of the lumbar vertebrae and the iliacus on the internal surface of the ilium. These two unite and attach distally to the lesser trochanter of the femur. This is a powerful flexor at the hip; especially when the knee is extended.

Discrepancy exists as to whether the *pectineus* (D) (color sky blue) should be listed with the anterior or medial thigh muscle groups. This muscle functions as both a flexor and an adductor of the thigh: thus the confusion. As you will learn in a future lesson this muscle is usually innervated by nerves supplying both the anterior (flexor) and medial (adductor) muscle groups.

The *tensor fascia latae* (E) (color blue) is the most anterior of the muscles on the lateral surface of the ilium, attaching proximally from the area of the anterior superior iliac spine and distally into the iliotibial tract, a tough connective tissue band destined to reach the lateral condyle of the tibia. This muscle pulls on the iliotibial tract counteracting the tension of the gluteus maximus and steadying the trunk on the thigh and leg.

❓ FOR REVIEW AND THOUGHT

The strength of the quadriceps femoris is crucial to performance in athletics as well as the quality of everyday locomotion! Why?

List several life or sport activities/skills requiring flexion at the hip with the knee kept extended.

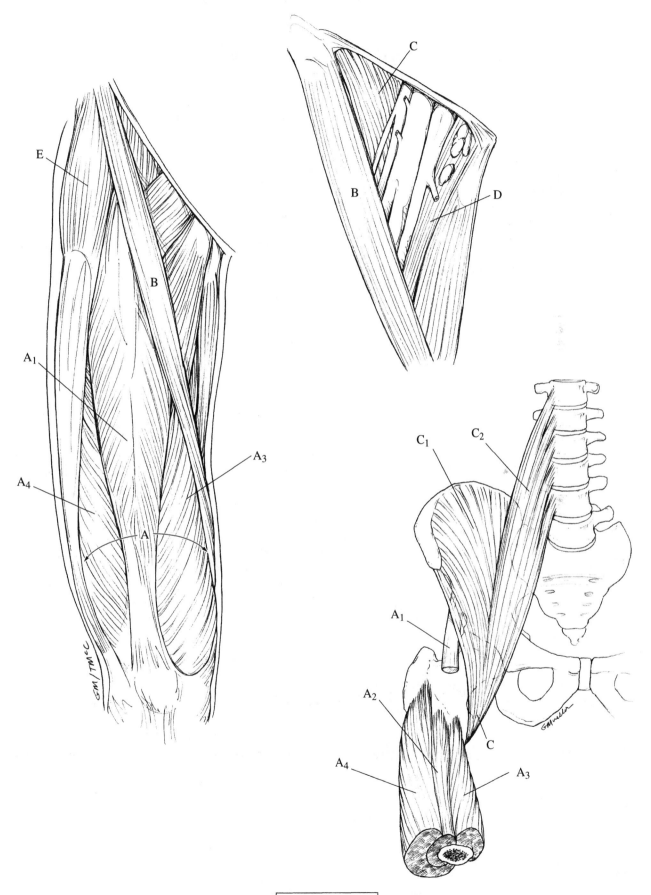

FIGURE 11.2

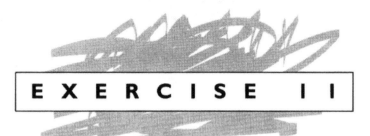

Muscles of the Lower Limb

POSTERIOR THIGH

The muscles of the posterior thigh are often called the 'hamstrings' in recognition of how hams were hung for smoking, by the stringy tendons of the posterior limb of the pig. In our discussion of these muscles we need to establish a definition of a true hamstring muscle. **A true hamstring has a proximal attachment off the ischial tuberosity and distal attachment to the tibia or fibula: thereby functioning at both the hip (extension) and knee (flexion).** With this definition established let's get on with the study of the posterior thigh (FIGURE 11.3).

The most lateral muscle of this group is the *biceps femoris* (A): composed of *long* (A₁) (color yellow) and *short* (A₂) (color orange) heads. The long head attaches proximally to the ischial tuberosity while the short head takes its attachment from the lateral lip of the linea aspera. The two heads join in one muscle belly attaching distally to the head of the fibula. **Given what you have just learned which head of the biceps femoris is a true hamstring?**

The *semitendinosus* (B) (color red-orange) also has a proximal attachment from the ischial tuberosity. Distally it attaches to the medial condyle of the tibia, somewhat anteriorly, via a long slender tendon. The final hamstring, *semimembranosus* (C) (color red) also takes proximal attachment from the ischial tuberosity. It attaches distally on the medial condyle of the tibia.

The tendons of these muscles are easily palpated while sitting with the knee flexed to 90°. With your fingers follow the tendon of the biceps femoris to its attachment on the head of the fibula. On the medial side of the popliteal region the tendon of the semitendinosus is equally palpable, although a little more difficult to follow completely to its tibial attachment. Just deep and medial to this tendon is the belly of the semimembranosus.

A fourth muscle, the *adductor magnus* (D) (color yellow-green), functions in part like a hamstring. This muscle, like the pectineus in the anterior thigh, may be described with two groups: posterior (extensor) and medial (adductor). Like the pectineus, it is innervated by two nerves; one for each group. A portion of the adductor magnus takes proximal attachment off the ischial tuberosity and descends the thigh to attach distally to the adductor tubercle of the medial epicondyle of the femur; thus not crossing the knee!

The medial collateral ligament of the knee is considered by some to be the antiquitous continuation of the adductor magnus. Such an explanation would also define this muscle as part hamstring.

❓ FOR REVIEW AND THOUGHT

You have probably heard of a "pulled hamstring muscle." Given what you have just learned about the muscles,

and keeping in mind the definition of a true hamstring, describe situations which might bring about such an injury!

MEDIAL THIGH

The medial compartment of the thigh contains five muscles: adductor magnus (already described in part with the posterior thigh), adductor longus, adductor brevis, pectineus (described in part with the anterior thigh), and the gracilis.

The 'adductor portion' of the *adductor magnus* (D) has proximal attachment off the ischial ramus and a portion of the inferior ramus of the pubis. Distal attachment is along the length of the medial ridge of the linea aspera. The magnus is a powerful adductor and is especially active in crossing the legs. The *adductor longus* (E) (color green) is the most anteriorly placed of the adductors. It takes proximal attachment from the body of the pubis just inferior to the pubic tubercles and attaches distally to the middle third of the medial lip of the linea aspera. *Adductor brevis* (F) (color sky blue) is found deep to the longus and pectineus. It takes proximal attachment from the body and inferior ramus of the pubis and distal attachment on the pectineal line and the superior third of the medial lip of the linea aspera. The *pectineus* (G) (color sky blue) passes from the pecten of the pubis as far as the pubic tubercle to a distal attachment on the pectineal line and proximal linea aspera.

The *gracilis* (H) (color blue) is just what its name implies graceful and delicate. It differs from other members of the medial thigh in shape, course, and function. This long slender muscle takes proximal attachment from the body of the pubis and is the only muscle of the adductor group to function at two joints. Distal attachment is on the anteromedial surface of the proximal tibia.

☾ JUST FOR FUN

Three muscles (sartorius, semitendinosus, and gracilis), from three different compartments of the thigh (anterior, posterior, and medial) attach distally in a small area of the anteromedial aspect of the tibia: **the pes anserine!** Named after the resemblance to the foot of a goose! Describe the functions of each of these muscles at the hip and at the knee.

Work with a partner and describe the functions of all the muscles we have studied in the three compartments of the thigh. Be especially aware of two-joint muscles and those with more than one function at a joint (*examples: semimembranosus, pectineus*)!

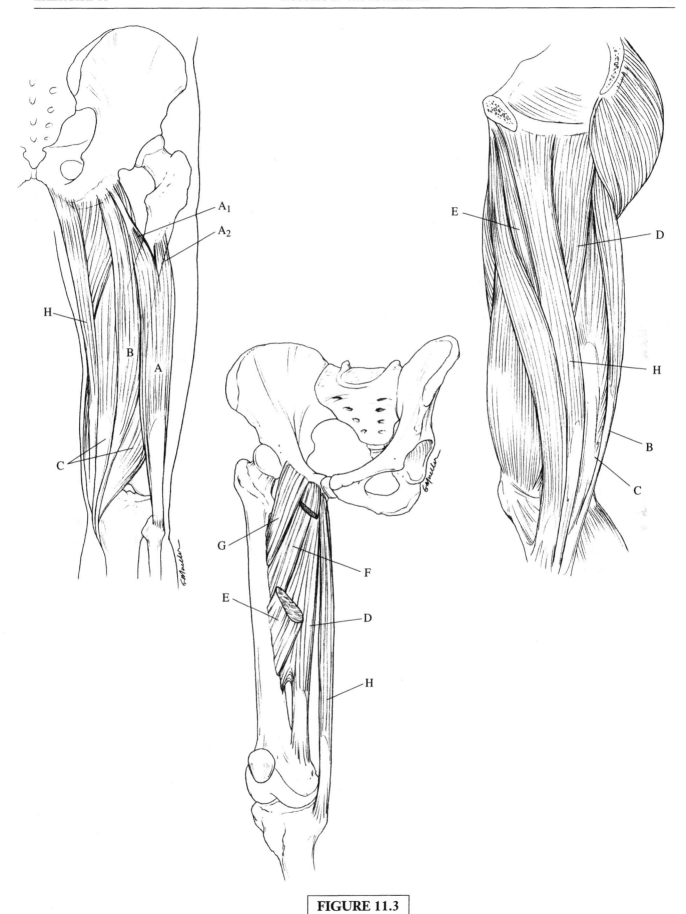

FIGURE 11.3

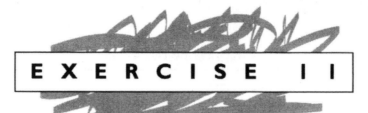

EXERCISE 11

Muscles of the Lower Limb

LEG

The leg is also divided nicely into three compartments, each with its own nerve. An interosseous membrane between the tibia and fibula separates the anterior (extensor) and posterior (flexor) compartments of the leg. The lateral (peroneal) compartment is the smallest and is bordered by anterior and posterior fascial septa passing deeply from the crural fascia and attaching to the fibula.

Two specific terms are used to describe movements at the talocrural joint: dorsi and plantar flexion. Dorsi flexion is the movement of the dorsal surface of the foot and the anterior surface of the leg toward one another (ex. assuming a squat position like a catcher in baseball). Plantar flexion is the opposite movement (ex. the catcher getting up on the heads of the metatarsals in anticipation of catching the pitch and continuing such movement in an attempt to throw out a base stealer). Inversion (turning in) and eversion (turning out) of the foot occur at the joints between the calcaneus and cuboid and the talus and navicular: the 'transverse tarsal joint' (see page 46).

ANTERIOR LEG

The *tibialis anterior* (A) (color yellow) (FIGURE 11.4) takes attachment from the lateral surface of the tibia, interosseous membrane, and the crural fascia. Its tendon passes into the foot, bound by superior and inferior extensor retinacula, to attach to the plantar surface of the medial cuneiform and the first metatarsal. This muscle is a dorsi flexor of the foot.

The interosseus membrane and medial surface of the fibula give proximal attachment to the *extensor hallucis longus* (B) (color orange). Attachment on the distal phalanx of the great toe is achieved via a tendon that passes beneath the retinacula.

Extensor digitorum longus (C) (color red-orange) has a somewhat similar course. From a proximal attachment on the lateral condyle of the tibia, shaft of the fibula, and interosseus membrane it passes deep to the retinacula, splits into four tendons, and reaches the distal phalanx of digits 2-5. This muscle sometimes has another tendon associated with it that passes to the dorsal surface of the fifth metatarsal. If present this extra tendon may even have a separate proximal attachment from the distal third of the fibula, and is called the *peroneus tertius* (D) (color red).

☺ JUST FOR FUN

What is the function of the retinacula?

LATERAL LEG

Peroneus is derived from the Latin word for fibula and describes the proximal attachment of both muscles in this compartment. The *peroneus longus* (E) (color yellow-green) has a proximal attachment off the head and proximal one-third of the fibula. The tendon of this muscle passes posterior to the lateral malleolus of the fibula and across the plantar surface of the foot, to an attachment on the base of the first metatarsal and medial cuneiform. It is a powerful everter of the foot as well as a plantar flexor. It is this tendon that causes the groove on the inferior surface of the cuboid bone (see page 16). The *peroneus brevis* (F) (color green) is like a younger sibling: it tries to do the same thing but only succeeds partially! After taking proximal attachment off the shaft of the fibula it too passes posterior to the lateral malleolus to reach its distal attachment on the tuberosity of the fifth metatarsal. It is a plantar flexor but a much weaker everter than the longus.

POSTERIOR LEG

The superficial layer of muscles includes the 'triceps surae' (three-headed muscle of the calf) composed of the *gastrocnemius* (G) (color sky blue) and *soleus* (H) (color blue). A third muscle, the *plantaris* (I) (color violet) is not always present and is a very weak player in any case. The gastrocnemius takes proximal attachment via two heads from the posterior surface of the femoral condyles and the soleus from the upper third of the fibula and tibia. The tendons of these muscles join as the calcaneal (Achilles) tendon for distal attachment on the tuber calcanei. The plantaris has a proximal attachment off the lateral femoral condyle and a distal on the tuber calcanei just medial to the calcaneal tendon. The triceps surae is a powerful plantar flexor of the foot. In addition the gastrocnemius, by virtue of its proximal attachment superior and posterior to the knee joint is also a flexor at the knee (free limb) and an accessory extensor at the knee (weight-bearing limb).

The deep group of muscles acts more distally, just as was the case in the upper limb. The *tibialis posterior* (J) (color light brown) has a proximal attachment from the posterior surface of the tibia, fibula, and intervening interosseus membrane. Its tendon passes posterior to the medial malleolus to reach the plantar surface of the navicular and cuneiform bones and the bases of metatarsals 2, 3, and 4. This muscle is a powerful plantar flexor. Two other muscles: *flexor digitorum longus* (K) (color brown) and *flexor hallucis longus* (L) (color black) have proximal attachment from the posterior surface of the tibia. The tendon of each passes posterior to the medial malleolus to find distal attachment: the flexor hallucis to the terminal phalanx of the first digit and the flexor digitorum to the terminal phalanges of digits 2-5. All of these muscles assist in plantar flexion at the ankle.

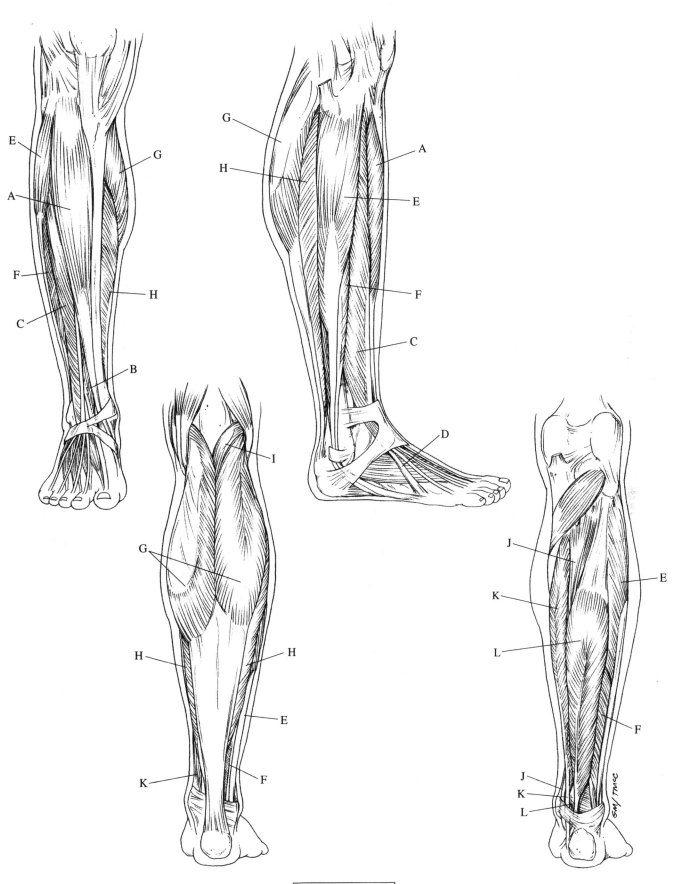

FIGURE 11.4

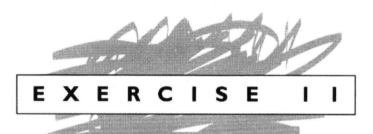

EXERCISE 11

Muscles of the Lower Limb

❓ FOR REVIEW AND THOUGHT

Take a few minutes to review the muscles of the leg. Which are involved in plantar flexion? What do all of these muscles have in common? What do all the dorsi flexors have in common?

MUSCLES OF THE FOOT

The intrinsic muscles of the foot (FIGURE 11.5) are organized in a fashion similar to those of the hand. As with the hand the specificity of function is greater on the plantar surface. This is so because more intrinsic muscles are found on the plantar surface than on the dorsal. Most of the dorsum of the foot is occupied by the tendons of the extrinsic muscles of the anterior compartment of the leg. These tendons are held in place by the extensor retinaculum. The one intrinsic muscle to be found is the *extensor digitorum brevis* (A) (color yellow). The belly of this muscle comes from the anterior surface of the calcaneus. It splits into three tendons to digits 2, 3, and 4 that attach via a dorsal aponeurosis. This muscle is responsible for dorsiflexion of these digits. A small *extensor hallucis brevis* (B) (color orange) splits off from the extensor digitorum brevis to pass to the first metatarsal. It too is a dorsiflexor.

The muscles of the plantar surface are more numerous and are arranged in layers. All are deep to a dense and tough plantar aponeurosis derived from the superficial fascia of the foot. The first layer includes the *abductor hallucis, flexor digitorum brevis, and abductor digiti minimi.* The function of these muscles is obvious from their name. Knowing only this into what phalanx of the toes would you expect the tendons of flexor digitorum brevis to attach?

In the first layer of the plantar surface the *abductor hallucis* (C) (color red-orange) attaches proximally on the medial side of the tuber calcanei and the plantar aponeurosis. Its tendon attaches distally into the medial sesamoid bone of the first metatarsal and the proximal phalanx. *Flexor digitorum brevis* (D) (color red) passes from the underside of the tuber calcanei and the deep surface of the plantar aponeurosis to form four tendons attaching into the middle phalanx of digits 2-5. Near their termination these tendons split (some authors describe this muscle as flexor digitorum perforatus) and the tendons of flexor digitorum longus pass through these gaps to reach the distal phalanges of the digits. Seem familiar? In what context have you already seen this?

Abductor digiti minimi (E) (color yellow-green) is the largest muscle of the little digit. Its attachments are the lateral surface of the tuber calcanei and the base of the proximal phalanx of digit 5.

The occupants of the second layer are both important players in the foot. The *quadratus plantae* (F) (color green), also known as the flexor accessorius, passes from the plantar surface of the calcaneus to the common tendon of the *flexor digitorum longus* (G) (color sky blue). Can you anticipate the roles of these two muscles? The flexor digitorum longus contracts and the quadratus plantae responds to correct the medial deviation that would occur due to the angle at which the flexor digitorum longus tendon passes through the foot!

The third layer of the plantar foot includes four *lumbricals* (H) (color blue) organized in much the same manner as those in the hand, except they pass from the medial side of each tendon of the flexor digitorum longus! Why this difference? Return briefly to page 66 to study the lumbricals of the hand and keep in mind the anatomical position and the differing roles of the hands and feet!

This layer also includes the *adductor hallucis* (I) (color violet) comprised of oblique and transverse heads, the *flexor hallucis brevis* (J), the *flexor digiti minimi* (K), and the *opponens digiti minimi* (L). Compare the positions and attachments of these muscles with their counterparts in the hand.

The deepest layer of the foot contains the interosseus muscles. Three *plantar* (M) (color light brown) and four *dorsal interossei* (N) (color brown) are present, as was the case with the hand. The line about which abduction and adduction is defined is the middle of the second digit. What was it in the hand?

❓ FOR REVIEW AND THOUGHT

You have now learned the muscles of the upper and lower limbs. For your conceptual understanding try to picture 'equivalent' muscles from these limbs. Don't be simplistic!

Upper Limb	Lower Limb
Deltoid	_____
_____	Plantaris
Fl. digitorum profundus	_____
_____	Piriformis
Adductor pollicis	_____
_____	Adductor magnus
Triceps brachii	_____
_____	Tibialis posterior

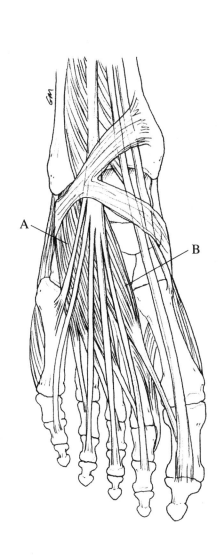

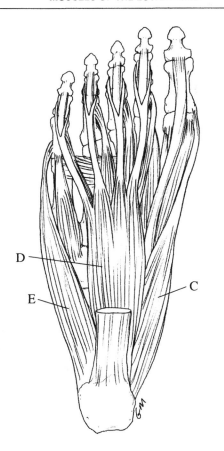

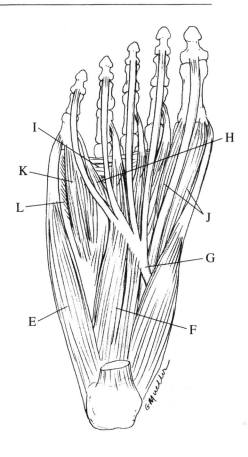

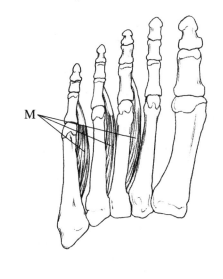

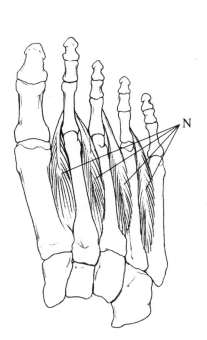

FIGURE 11.5

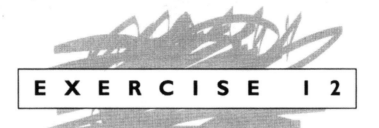

Muscles of the Trunk and Neck

INTRINSIC MUSCLES OF THE BACK

This group of muscles (collectively referred to as the *erector spinae*) is innervated segmentally by dorsal primary rami of spinal nerves. These are, indeed, muscles of the back and function in maintaining the upright stance against gravity. It is not our intention to describe and discuss every muscle, but rather to focus on the function of the group as a whole (FIGURE 12.1).

As a unit the erector spinae sweep from the sacrum to the skull. This unit has three major subdivisions: iliocostalis, longissimus, and spinalis and each of these, in turn, has three portions. The most lateral subdivision is the *iliocostalis* (A) (color yellow). Its three portions are *lumborum* (A_1), *thoracis* (A_2), and *cervicis* (A_3). The iliocostalis lumborum extends from the sacrum to the inferior six to nine ribs, the thoracis from the inferior six to the superior six ribs, and the cervicis from ribs 6 to 3 to the transverse processes of cervical vertebra 4-6.

The second subdivision, the *longissimus* (B) (color orange), includes the *thoracis* (B_1) portion from the sacrum and spinous processes of the lumbar vertebrae to the first or second ribs; the *cervicis* (B_2), passing from the transverse processes of the upper six thoracic vertebrae to the posterior tubercles of the transverse processes of cervical vertebra 2-5; and the *capitis* (B_3), from the transverse processes of T_{1-3} and C_{5-7} to the mastoid processes of the temporal bones of the skull.

The *spinalis* (C) (color red-orange) is the most medial of the three subdivisions. The *thoracis* (C_1) extends from the spinous processes of L_3-T_{10} to the spinous processes of T_{8-2} vertebra; the *cervicis* (C_2) passes from spinous processes of T_2-C_6 to the spinous processes of C_{4-2}. The most superior portion, *capitis* (C_3), is seldom present.

In these descriptions did you notice we passed from lateral to medial: iliocostalis – longissimus – spinalis, between groups; and inferior to superior: lumborum – thoracis – cervicis – capitis, within groups? It is important to keep this concept of the erector spinae in mind: a functional muscle mass from sacrum to skull with the task of maintaining upright posture against the constant force of gravity!

Several other muscles of the back and neck require description. Deep to the erector spinae are smaller muscles functioning between only one or two vertebral levels. The *rotatores brevis* (D) (color red) and *longus* (E) (color yellow-green) are most prominent in the thoracic region. Each takes proximal attachment from a transverse process and passes to the first (brevis) or second (longus) spinous process above. The *multifidi* (F) (color green) are small muscles found from the sacrum to the 2nd cervical verte-bra. Each passes from the aponeurosis of the longissimus and ascends two to four vertebral levels to attach distally on a spinous process.

Two muscle groups remain to be described: semispinalis and splenius. The *semispinalis* (G) is superficial to the multifidi and is divided into thoracic, cervical, and capital portions. *Semispinalis thoracis* (G_1) (color sky blue) and *cervicis* (G_2) (color blue) have proximal attachment from the transverse processes of all thoracic vertebrae and attach distally to the spinous processes of the superior six thoracic and inferior four cervical vertebrae. These muscles extend the thoracic and cervical regions of the column. *Semispinalis capitis* (G_3) (color violet) passes from the transverse processes of the superior 4-7 thoracic vertebrae and the articular processes of the five inferior cervical vertebra to the skull; attaching between the superior and inferior nuchal lines. This muscle functions in extension of the head.

The *splenius cervicis* (H) (color light brown) courses from the spinous processes of the 3rd through 6th thoracic vertebrae to the transverse processes of the 1st and 2nd cervical vertebrae. The *splenius capitis* (I) (color brown) has proximal attachment from the superior three thoracic and inferior four cervical vertebrae and distal attachment on the lateral portion of the superior nuchal line and the mastoid process of the temporal bone. Acting on one side only these muscles laterally rotate and flex the head toward that side. Acting together these muscles extend the neck.

❓ FOR REVIEW AND THOUGHT

What is the general function of the erector spinae?

Having answered this how would you describe the relationship of proximal and distal attachments of these muscles?

What is the nerve supply of the erector spinae and does it differ in any way from that of the limb muscles?

🕚 JUST FOR FUN

When you were a youth your parents may have told you many times to "sit up straight" or "stand tall," usually in response to you slouching or looking down at your feet. Were they referring to your 'erector spinae' in such exhortations or to muscles of the shoulder girdle located on the back?

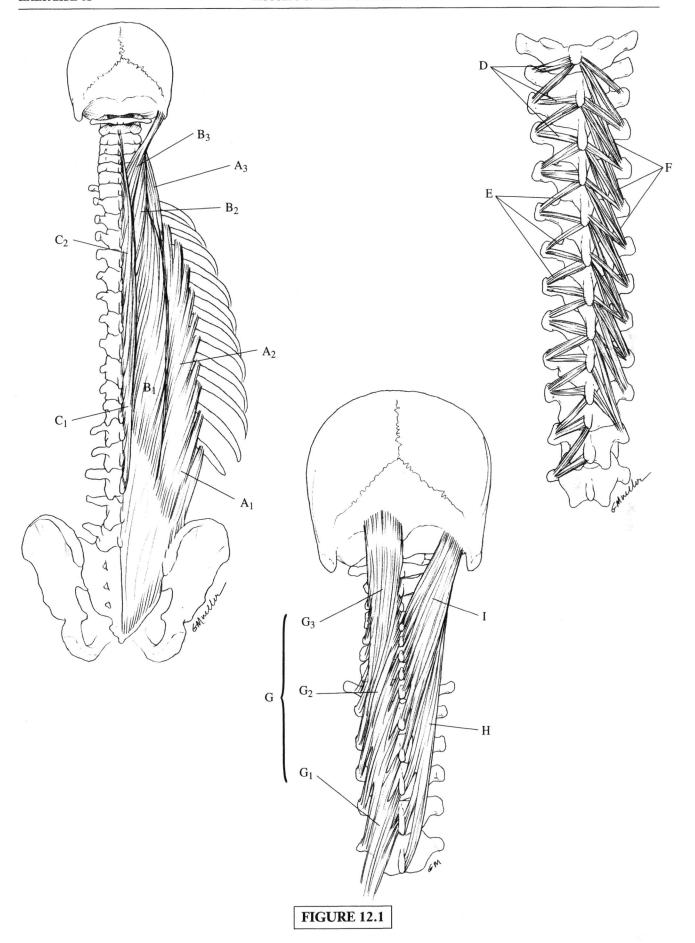

FIGURE 12.1

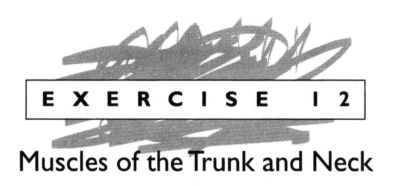

Muscles of the Trunk and Neck

MUSCLES OF RESPIRATION

The musculotendinous *diaphragm* (A) (color yellow) (FIGURE 12.2) is the primary muscle of respiration. It delineates the thorax (superior) from the abdomen (inferior). Its thoracic and abdominal surfaces are covered with parietal pleura and parietal peritoneum respectively. When contracted the volume of the thoracic cavity is increased, aiding inspiration. When relaxed just the opposite occurs: thoracic volume is decreased, aiding in expiration.

The area between each pair of ribs is an intercostal space and there are, therefore, eleven such spaces. Each intercostal space contains three muscles arranged in incomplete layers. The most superficial is the *external intercostal* (B) (color orange), observable in the midlateral portion of the intercostal space with fibers passing inferiorly and medially from the rib above to the one below. In the more inferior intercostal spaces this muscle is continuous with the external oblique muscle of the abdomen. In the midline, as these muscles approach the costal cartilages, they are replaced by the external intercostal membrane.

The *internal intercostal* (C) (color red-orange) muscles course at right angles (superiorly and medially) to the external. From the angle of the rib to the vertebrae this layer is replaced by the internal intercostal membrane. The deepest layer is the *innermost intercostals* (D) (color red). These fibers course in the same direction as those of the internal intercostal and between these two layers pass the intercostal arteries, veins, and nerves. *Subcostal* (E) (color yellow-green) muscles are variable in size and number

and are most often found in the inferior thorax. They often cross two intercostal spaces. The *transverse thoracis* muscles (F) are found on the deep surface of the sternum passing to costal cartilages 2-6. The twelve pair of *levatores costarum* (G) take proximal attachment on the transverse processes of C_7-T_{11}. Distally they attach between the tubercle and angle of the rib below. They elevate the ribs during respiration.

ACCESSORY MUSCLES OF RESPIRATION

Muscles other than those already described play a role in respiration. The *serratus posterior superior* (H) has its proximal attachment on the spinous processes of the last two cervical and first two thoracic vertebrae and distal attachment on the angles of ribs 2-5. It functions to elevate these ribs; therefore aiding in inspiration. The *serratus posterior inferior* (I) takes proximal attachment off the spinous processes of T_{11}-L_2 and distal attachment on the inferior border of ribs 9-12, near their angles. It fixes these ribs; also aiding in inspiration.

Three other muscles act as aids to respiration. The *scalenus anterior* (J) takes proximal attachment from the anterior tubercles of cervical vertebrae 3-6 and distal attachment on the first rib. The *scalenus medius* (K) passes from the posterior tubercles of cervical vertebrae 2-7 to the superior surface of the first rib. The *scalenus posterior* (L) courses from the posterior tubercles of cervical vertebrae 4-6 to the second rib. These muscles function to elevate the first two ribs and are critical in quiet respiration.

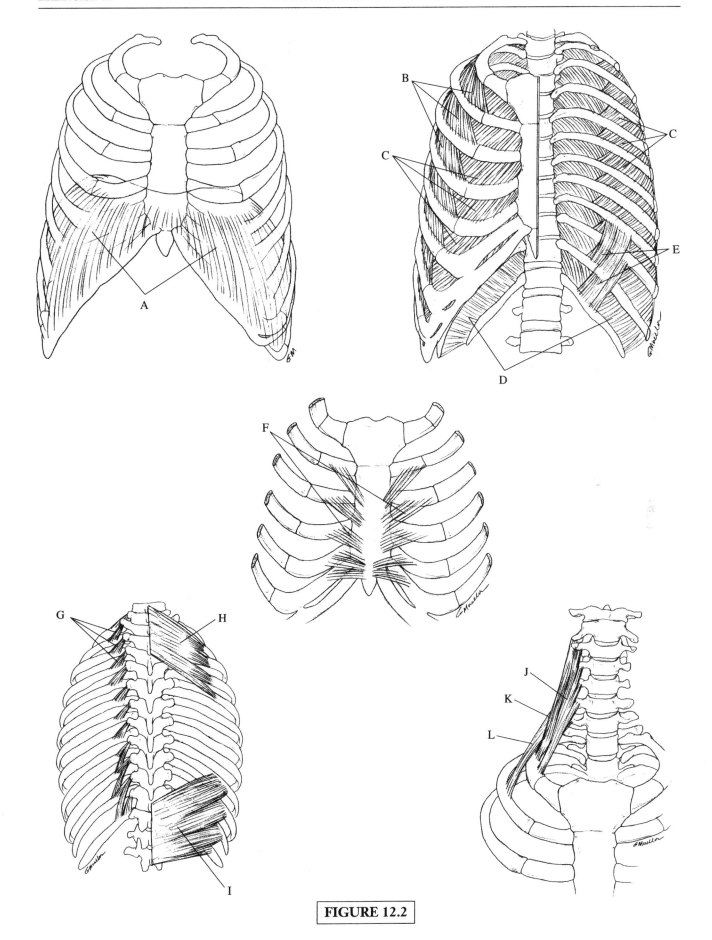

FIGURE 12.2

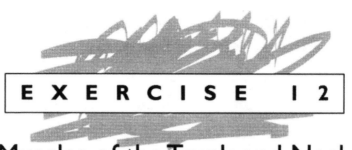

Muscles of the Trunk and Neck

ABDOMINAL MUSCLES

The anterolateral wall of the abdomen (FIGURE 12.3) is formed by four muscles; three of them lateral and one anterior. The *rectus abdominus* (A) (color green) is prominent in the midline. This paired muscle passes from its proximal attachment on the pubic crest and symphysis to the anterior surface of the xiphoid process and of the costal cartilages of ribs 5-7. Between the two halves of the rectus a tough midline structure, the *linea alba* (B), is found. Enclosing the muscle is the *rectus sheath* (C), formed by the aponeurotic extensions of the three lateral muscles of the abdomen. The anterior layer of this sheath is firmly bound to the rectus at several points: the *tendinous intersections* (D). The 'ripped' appearance of the rectus when well developed owes to these tendinous intersections! The rectus abdominus functions in flexion of the trunk.

The aponeurotic portions of the other three muscles also contribute to the rectus sheath. The *external oblique* (E) (color sky blue) is the most superficial of these muscles; passing inferomedially from the external surfaces of the 5th to 12th ribs to a distal attachment on the iliac crest and the anterior surface of the rectus sheath. Deep to the external oblique is the *internal oblique* (F) (color blue) with fibers running at a right angles (superomedial) to those of the external. The proximal attachment of this muscle is from the iliac crest and inguinal ligament. Distally it attaches to the cartilages of ribs 10-12 and the aponeurosis of the rectus sheath. The *transverse abdominus* (G) (color violet) is the deepest of the three layered muscles of the abdominal wall. It takes proximal attachment off the deep surfaces of the costal cartilages of ribs 7-12. Its fibers pass transversely to attach in the deep surface in the rectus sheath. These muscles function to regulate intraabdominal pressure and are active in forced expiration.

One final muscle requires description. The paired *quadratus lumborum* (H) (color brown) take proximal attachment from the posterior portion of the iliac crest and distal attachment on the transverse processes of lumbar vertebrae 1-4 and the 12th rib. Acting singly each is a lateral flexor of the trunk. Acting together they stabilize, and perhaps slightly depress, the 12th rib.

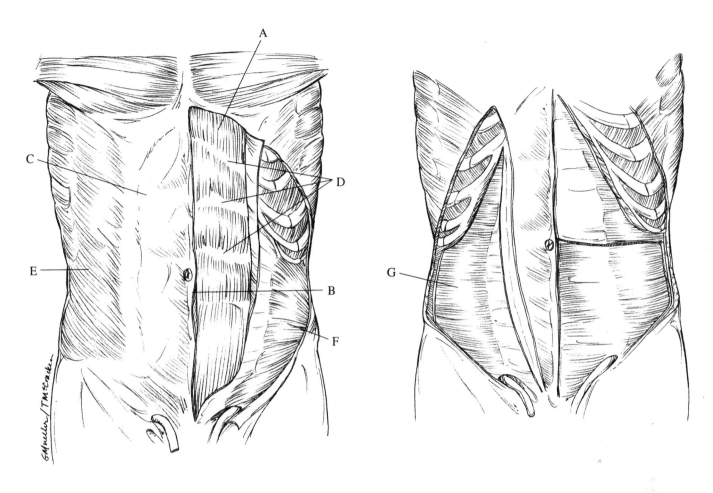

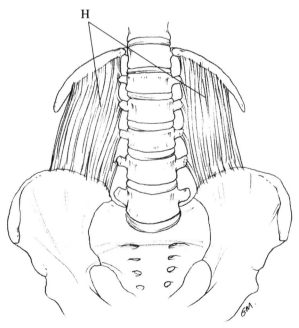

FIGURE 12.3

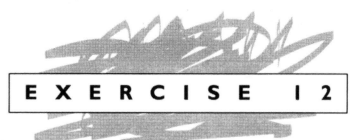

EXERCISE 12

Muscles of the Trunk and Neck

PELVIC MUSCULATURE

The pelvic cavity is merely an extension of the abdominal cavity with no obvious border. The pelvis (L., basin) is conceptually divided into false and ture portions. The false pelvis is immediately continuous with the abdomen and is the area superior to the pelvic inlet; protected by the wings of the ilia. The true pelvis is inferior to the inlet and is bounded laterally and inferiorly by a muscular diaphragm which serves to close the pelvic outlet. The paired muscles involved in this are the *levatores ani* (A) and *coccygeus* (B) (FIGURE 12.4).

The levator ani are the more important of the two portions of the diaphragm. The fibers of the muscle have proximal attachment off the pubis anteriorly and from the fascia of the *obturator internus* (C) (color green) laterally. This is called the *tendinous arc of the levator ani* (D). The muscle is divided into three portions: the *pubococcygeus* (A$_1$) (color yellow), *puborectalis* (A$_2$) (color orange), and *iliococcygeus* (A$_3$) (color red-orange). In the midline the fibers of this muscle interlock and attach partially into the structures piercing the diaphragm, thus providing support and possibly some control.

The fibers of the *coccygeus* muscle (color red) fan out from the ischial spine to attach to the lateral surface of the sacrum and coccyx. The *piriformis* (E) muscle (color blue) closes the remainder of the pelvic bowl posteriorly. This muscle takes proximal attachment off the anterior surface of the sacrum and passes to the greater trochanter of the femur.

A frontal section of this area provides a clear image of the bowl formed by the levator ani and the position of the obturator internus. This muscle, plus its external counterpart and the obturator membrane nearly completely seal the obturator foramen (see Active Learning, page 10).

❓ FOR REVIEW AND THOUGHT

What structures pierce the pelvic diaphragm?

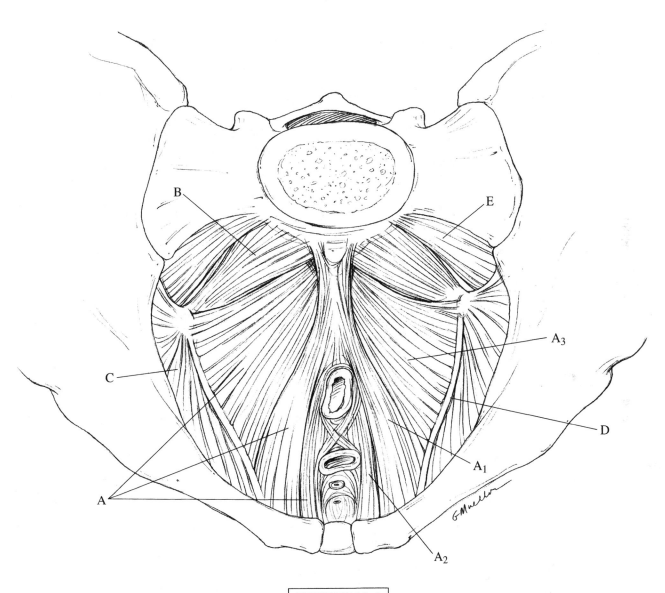

FIGURE 12.4

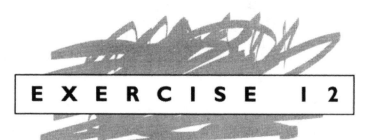

EXERCISE 12

Muscles of the Trunk and Neck

SUPERFICIAL

The neck is geographically divided into triangles with specific boundaries (FIGURE 12.5). The two main divisions are the *anterior* (A) and *posterior* (B) triangles. The anterior triangle is bounded medially by the cervical midline, laterally by the sternocleidomastoid muscle, and superiorly by the body of the mandible (outline this triangle in yellow). The subdivisions of this triangle are as follows:

submandibular (A₁) – bounded by the bellies of the digastric muscle posteriorly and by the body of the mandible anteriorly (outline in orange)

carotid (A₂) – bounded by the sternocleidomastoid posteriorly, the superior belly of the omohyoid muscle anteriorly, and the posterior belly of the digastric superiorly (outline in red-orange)

muscular (A₃) – bounded by the cervical midline medially, by the superior belly of the omohyoid superolaterally, and by the sternocleidomastoid inferolaterally (outline in red)

submental (A₄) – bounded medially by the cervical midline, by the anterior belly of the digastric laterally, and by the hyoid bone inferiorly (outline in yellow-green)

The *posterior triangle* (B) is bounded by the trapezius posteriorly, the sternocleidomastoid anteriorly, and the clavicle inferiorly (outline this triangle in sky blue). The posterior triangle is subdivided as follows:

occipital (B₁) – bounded anteriorly and posteriorly as described above and inferiorly by the posterior belly of the omohyoid (outline in blue)

omoclavicular (B₂) – bounded anteriorly by the sternocleidomastoid, superiorly by the posterior belly of the omohyoid, and inferiorly by the clavicle (outline in violet)

Perhaps the key muscle in the neck is the *sternocleidomastoid* (C) (color brown). It takes proximal attachment off the manubrium of the sternum and the medial third of the clavicle and passes to the mastoid process of the temporal bone for distal attachment. Working with its mate on the opposite side it produces flexion of the head. Working singly it elevates the chin and rotates the head to the opposite side.

Three 'straplike' muscles: *sternohyoid* (D) (color yellow), *sternothyroid* (E) (color orange), and *thyrohyoid* (F) (color red-orange) are found in the anterior neck (FIGURE 12.5). The sternohyoid is superficial, with the other two deep to it. The proximal and distal attachments of these muscles should be obvious to you. Note that all of these are paired (bilateral). As a group they are called the infrahyoid strap muscles. What, then, would you consider the function of this group to be?

A muscle somewhat associated with these is the *omohyoid* (G) (color red) Deep to the sternocleidomastoid an intermediate tendon is connected to the clavicle by a fascial loop: dividing the omohyoid into inferior and superior bellies.

▶ ACTIVE LEARNING

Find the hyoid bone (called such, but actually cartilage) on yourself. To do this place your thumb and index finger on the angles of your mandible, tip up your chin, slide your thumb and finger anteriorly about 1½ inches, and press gently.

The two bellies of the *digastric* muscle (H) (color green) have disparate proximal attachments: the anterior belly from the digastric fossa on the deep surface of the mandible and the posterior belly from the mastoid notch of the temporal bone. These bellies have distal attachment on the greater cornu of the hyoid bone via a fibrous slip. This muscle elevates and steadies the hyoid bone in swallowing and speaking.

Other muscles with distal attachment on the hyoid bone include the *mylohyoid* (I) (color sky blue), *stylohyoid* (J) (color violet), and *geniohyoid* (K) (color light brown). All of these, along with the digastric, are suprahyoid muscles. These muscles have proximal attachment from the mylohyoid line on the deep surface of the mandible, the genoid tubercle of the mandible, and the styloid process of the temporal bone respectively.

Find your hyoid bone again and swallow. What happens to the hyoid bone when you do this? What would be the collective function of these muscles?

❓ FOR REVIEW AND THOUGHT

Place the muscles you have just learned in one (or more) triangles of the neck.

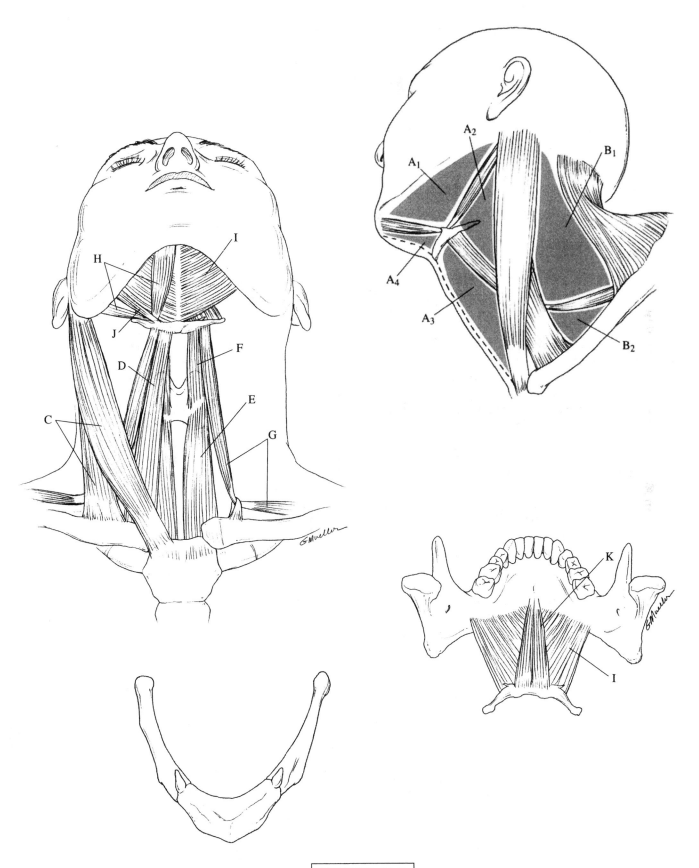

FIGURE 12.5

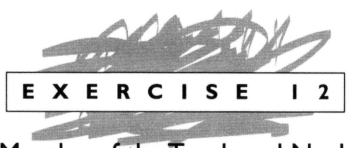

EXERCISE 12

Muscles of the Trunk and Neck

ANTERIOR VERTEBRAL

Four muscles are found on the anterior surface of the vertebral column (FIGURE 12.6a). All are described as prevertebral. As a group these four muscles function in flexion and rotation of the head.

The *longus colli* (A) spans the distance from T_3 vertebra to the atlas. It attaches in part to the bodies of all the intervening vertebrae and the transverse processes of C_{3-6}. An associated muscle, the *longus capitis* (B), takes proximal attachment from the anterior tubercles of the transverse processes of C_{3-6}. Its distal attachment is on the basilar portion of the occipital bone. Both of these muscles function in flexion and rotation of the cervical vertebrae and the head

Two very small muscles span the gap between the atlas and the base of the skull. The *rectus capitis anterior* (C) (color yellow) attaches proximally to the lateral mass of the atlas and distally to the base of the occipital bone anterior to the foramen magnum. Its companion, the *rectus capitis lateralis* (D) (color orange) courses from the transverse process of the atlas to the inferior surface of the jugular process of the occipital bone. These muscles function in flexion and rotation of the head on the neck.

SUBOCCIPITAL MUSCLES

Four small muscles are found deep in the posterior cervical region (FIGURE 12.6b). The *rectus capitis posterior major* (E) (color green) passes from the spinous process of the axis to the lateral portion of the inferior nuchal line of the occipital bone. It functions to rotate the head toward the same side as well as to extend the neck. The *rectus capitis posterior minor* (F) (color sky blue) has much the same course and function. It passes from the posterior tubercle of the atlas to the inferior nuchal line of the occipital bone. The *obliquus capitis inferior* (G) (color blue) passes from the spine of the axis to the transverse process of the atlas; producing rotation of the skull to its side. This muscle and its twin on the opposite side, contracting reciprocally, allow us to answer NO without speaking! The last small muscle of the region is the *obliquus capitis superior* (H) (color violet). From a proximal attachment on the transverse process of the atlas it runs superiorly and medially to a distal attachment on the occipital bone superior to the inferior nuchal line. It functions to flex the head laterally and posteriorly.

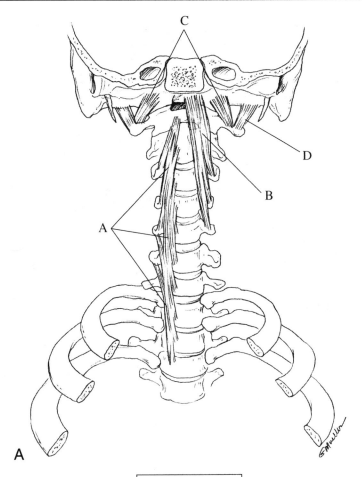

A

FIGURE 12.6a

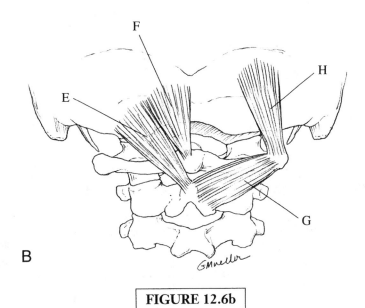

B

FIGURE 12.6b

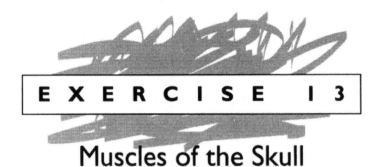

EXERCISE 13

Muscles of the Skull

MUSCLES OF MASTICATION

Four muscles of mastication (chewing) are described: temporalis, masseter, medial pterygoid, and lateral pterygoid (FIGURE 13.1). The *temporalis* (A) (color yellow) has a proximal attachment on the lateral surface of the frontal and temporal bones and a distal attachment on the coronoid process and anterior surface of the mandibular ramus. The *masseter* (B) (color orange) takes proximal attachment from the inferior edge and deep surface of the zygomatic arch and finds distal attachment on the lateral surface of the ramus and angle of the mandible. The *medial pterygoid* (C) (color red-orange) takes proximal attachment from two sites: a deep head from the medial surface of the pterygoid plate and a superficial head from the tuberosity of the maxilla. Distally this muscle attaches to the deep surface of the angle of the mandible. The *lateral pterygoid* (D) (color red) also has proximal attachment via two heads: one from the infratemporal ridge of the sphenoid bone (the upper head) and the lower head from the lateral surface of the lateral pterygoid plate. Distal attachment is found on the neck of the mandible.

In the process of mastication the temporalis, masseter, and medial pterygoid all aid in elevating (closing) the mouth. The deep portion of the masseter and the lateral pterygoid cooperate in protruding the chin and all four muscles function in grinding movements.

MUSCLES OF FACIAL EXPRESSION

These muscles are unique in that they have one, or both, of their attachments into skin rather than bone. All muscles of facial expression are innervated by the Facial Nerve (Cranial Nerve VII). An exhaustive listing of all of these is beyond our intent here but we will describe some we find interesting and fun! Keep in mind that these muscles literally express how you feel.

Let's begin with the *zygomaticus* (E) (color yellow-green). You have probably guessed one attachment already. The zygomatic arch provides proximal attachment and distal attachment is into the angle of the mouth. It draws the angle of the mouth posteriorly and superiorly. *It's the laughing muscle!* An ally to the zygomaticus is the *levator anguli oris* (F) (color green), the elevator of the angle of the mouth: *the smiling muscle!* It has proximal attachment from the maxilla and distal attachment at the angle of the mouth. The final member of this happy trio is the *risorius* (G) (color sky blue) taking proximal attachment from the fascia overlying the masseter and attaching to the skin at the angle of the mouth: *the grinning muscle!*

The *depressor anguli oris* (H) passes from the inferior margin of the mandible to the angle of the mouth, which it depresses, producing an expression of sadness or grief.

The *depressor labii inferioris* (I) courses from the mandible to the skin of the lower lip, also evoking sadness.

The *mentalis* (J) passes from the mandible to the skin of the chin. It produces a furrowed chin as an expression of doubt.

An expression of discontent is produced by the *levator labii superioris alaeque nasi* (K) (color blue). This muscle has a proximal attachment on the infraorbital margin and zygomatic bone and distal attachment into the skin of the upper lip and nasal wing. (As well as one of the great names in anatomy!)

The *procerus* (L) (color violet) passes from the dorsal surface of the nose to the skin of the forehead between the eyebrows. It produces a wrinkling of skin across the bridge of the nose and a menacing expression. In old age these folds may be permanent.

The *buccinator* (M) (color light brown) courses from the alveolar process of the mandible to the angle of the mouth. This muscle compresses the cheeks and expels air between the lips (whistling). It is described as an accessory muscle of mastication; acting to keep the bolus of food between the teeth. It produces an expression of satisfaction.

Muscles of the scalp constitute the *epicranius* (O) with anterior and posterior bellies and a tough tendon, the galea aponeurotica in between. This layer stretches from the forehead to the occipital region. The muscular portion is the *occipitofrontalis* (P) consisting, not surprisingly, of frontal and occipital bellies. The occipital belly has proximal attachment from the superior nuchal line while the frontal belly has no bony attachment, arising from the skin of the eyebrow and glabella. The epicranius, via its anterior belly produces wrinkling of the forehead and elevation of the eyebrows and upper eyelids: an expression of surprise or astonishment.

The *orbicularis oris* (Q) (color brown) is a complex sphincter muscle encircling the mouth and mixing with other facial muscles. It closes the mouth and plays a key roles in speech and mastication. It presents an expression of reserve.

Finally, the *orbicularis oculi* (R) (color black), consisting of orbital, palpebral, and lacrimal portions. The orbital portion is involved in firm closure of the eyelids, the palpebral in blinking and light closure of the lids, and the lacrimal in drawing the lids slightly medially. This muscle produces an expression of concern, shown by wrinkling of the skin lateral to the orbit. With aging these wrinkles persist as 'crows feet'.

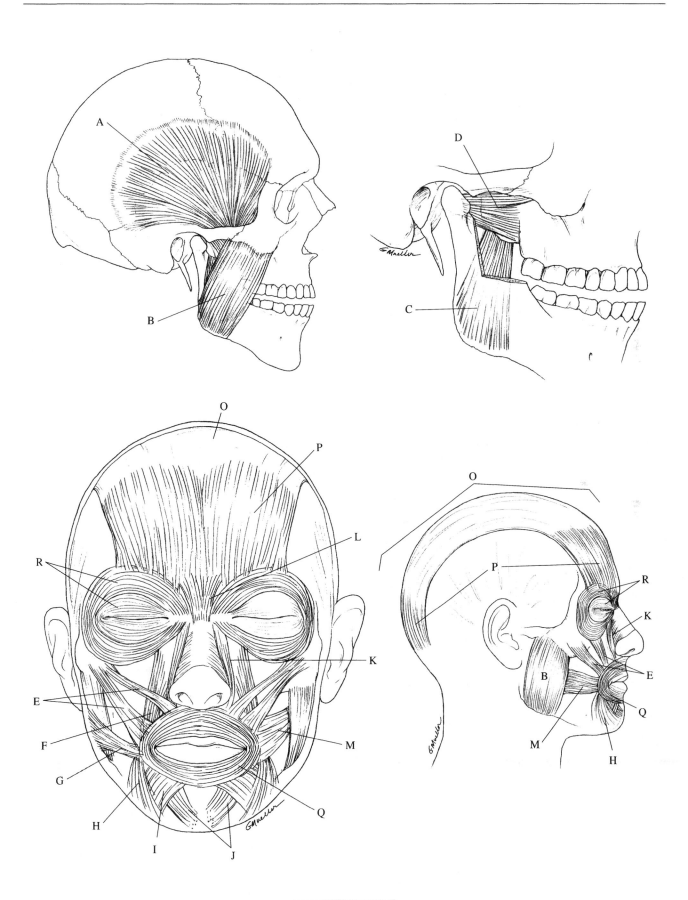

FIGURE 13.1

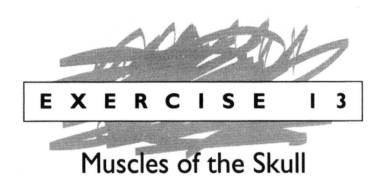

EXERCISE 13

Muscles of the Skull

EXTRAOCULAR MUSCLES

Seven muscles are found in the orbit. Six of these act to position the eyeball: four recti (straight) and two oblique, while the seventh elevates the superior eyelid. Let's begin with this muscle (FIGURE 13.2)!

The *levator palpebrae superioris* (A) (color yellow) has a proximal attachment off the orbital roof immediately anterior to the optic foramen. The distal attachment is via an aponeurotic sheath that spreads through the eyelid.

The four recti are specific in terminology and function. They elevate, depress, adduct, and abduct the eyeball. The oblique muscles aid in these functions as well as rotation of the eyeball.

The *medial rectus* (B) (color orange) has a proximal attachment, common to all the recti, from the annular tendon surrounding the margin of the optic foramen. It courses along the nasal wall of the orbit to find distal attachment into the sclera of the eyeball just posterior to the corneoscleral junction; producing adduction of the eyeball (movement toward the medial wall of the orbit). The *lateral rectus* (C) (color red-orange) passes along the temporal wall of the orbit and attaches similarly. It produces abduction of the eyeball.

The *superior* (D) (color green) and *inferior recti* (E) (color blue) pass from the annular tendon to their distal attachments, which are similar to that of the other recti. The superior elevates and the inferior depresses the eyeball.

The course taken by the oblique muscles is more complex resulting in increased functional abilities. The *superior oblique* (F) (color violet) courses from the annular tendon, along the medial wall of the orbit to pass through a fibrous ring, the *trochlea* (G). At this point the tendon re-verses direction to pass inferior to the superior rectus and attach via muscular fibers into the superior surface of the eyeball. This attachment is posterior to the transverse axis of the eyeball and lateral to the sagittal axis. Such attachments allow this muscle to abduct, depress, and internally rotate the eyeball.

The *inferior oblique muscle* (H) (color light brown) takes proximal attachment from the medial orbital floor, near the nasolacrimal duct, and passes laterally and posteriorly toward the temporal surface of the eyeball. Distal attachment is to the sclera between the lateral and superior recti posterior to the transverse axis and lateral to the sagittal axis. This muscle functions in abduction, elevation, and external rotation of the eyeball.

MUSCLES OF AUDITION

Two muscles are found in the middle ear. Each functions to enhance auditory reception. The *tensor tympani* (I) (color brown) courses from the cartilage of the auditory canal to the root of the handle of the malleus. Its name describes its function: a tensor of the tympanic membrane. The quite tiny *stapedius* (J) (color black) is found in the middle ear. It passes from the posterior wall of the tympanic cavity to the neck of the stapes. Contraction limits movement of the stapes thereby reducing oscillatory range.

❓ FOR REVIEW AND THOUGHT

List the six extraocular muscles with their actions on the eyeball and their innervations.

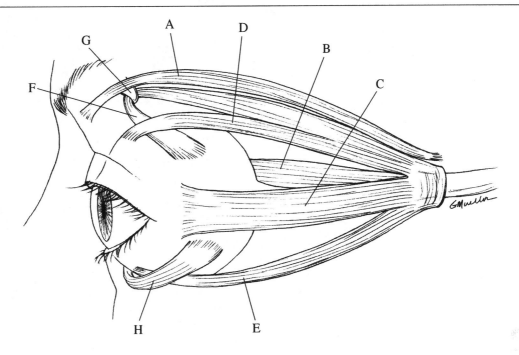

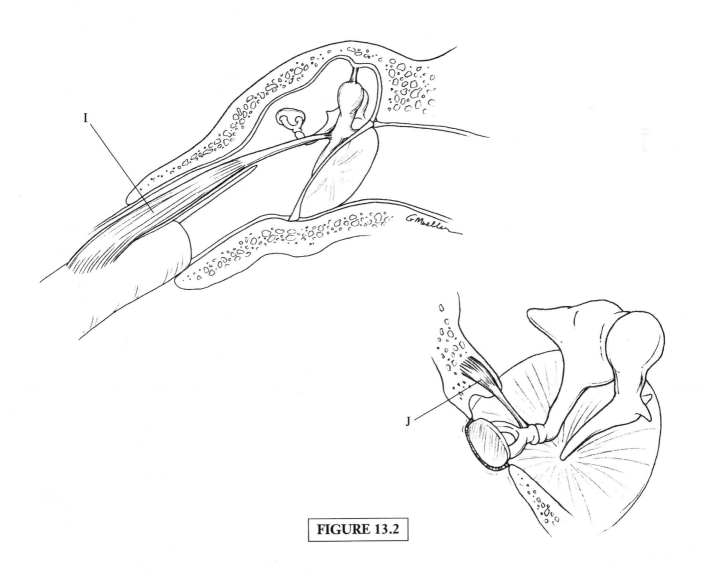

FIGURE 13.2

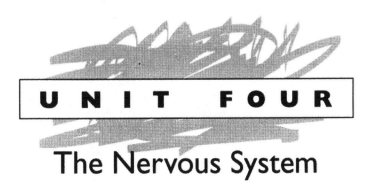

UNIT FOUR

The Nervous System

The nervous system serves the human in myriad ways from the depths of creative thought to the simple reflex arc; from the control of the heartbeat to the memories that come to us when 'oldies' are played on the radio; from sensations of pain to the feeling of pleasure; and the abilities to 'put the shot', 'tickle the ivories', 'dance Swan Lake', or reattach a human hand. A complete explanation of this system is not only beyond the scope of this text, but truly beyond learning.

The nervous system is compartmentalized as follows.

Central Nervous System (brain and spinal cord)
Peripheral Nervous System (nerves to the body wall and extremities)
Autonomic Nervous System (nerves to viscera), with Sympathetic and Parasympathetic portions

Since we have just completed study of the skeletal, articular, and muscular systems we will begin the investigation of the nervous system by learning the structure and function of the somatic portion of the peripheral nervous system. The basic structural unit of this portion is the **typical spinal nerve** (FIGURE IVa-c).

A typical spinal nerve involves a *dorsal root* (A) (color yellow) composed of sensory neurons and identified by the *dorsal root ganglion* (B), the site of the cell bodies of these neurons. The *ventral root* (C) (color orange) is composed of motor neurons from cell bodies located in the ventral horn of the spinal cord. Just prior to leaving the protection of the vertebral column these two roots join as the *spinal nerve* (D) (color red-orange), which almost immediately splits into a small *dorsal ramus* (E) (color red) and a larger *ventral ramus* (F) (color yellow-green). Dorsal rami will provide motor innervation to the erector spinae muscles and cutaneous sensory innervation to the overlying skin. Ventral rami are destined to innervate all other skeletal muscles and the remainder of the skin. The formation of a spinal nerve involves neurons with their cell bodies in a discrete geographic area of the spinal cord.

This organization of spinal nerves allows a mapping of sensory distribution known as dermatomes (FIGURE IVb,c). Each dermatome shows the areas of skin supplied by a pair of spinal nerves. The mapping of motor neuron distribution is somewhat less clear but nonetheless logical.

Three covering layers, known as *meninges*, surround the central nervous system. The outermost is the thickest and toughest, composed of connective tissue and intimately adherent to the inner surface of the cranium and vertebral column: *dura mater* (tough mother) (G). Deep to this lies the *arachnoid mater* (H), a delicate weblike layer beneath which lies the subarachnoid space containing cerebrospinal fluid. The deepest of the three meningeal layers, in intimate contact with the brain and spinal cord, is the *pia mater* (*gentle* mother) (I). This layer is highly vascularized. Denticulate ligaments (J), threadlike extensions of the pia matter, extend laterally in a rather routine manner.

All three meningeal layers continue along the spinal nerve as it exits the protection of the vertebral column at which point they fuse with the epineural covering of the spinal nerve. Each spinal nerve and its ventral and dorsal rami are mixed: carrying both motor and sensory neurons.

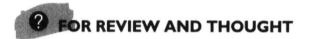

❓ FOR REVIEW AND THOUGHT

What are the component parts of a typical spinal nerve?

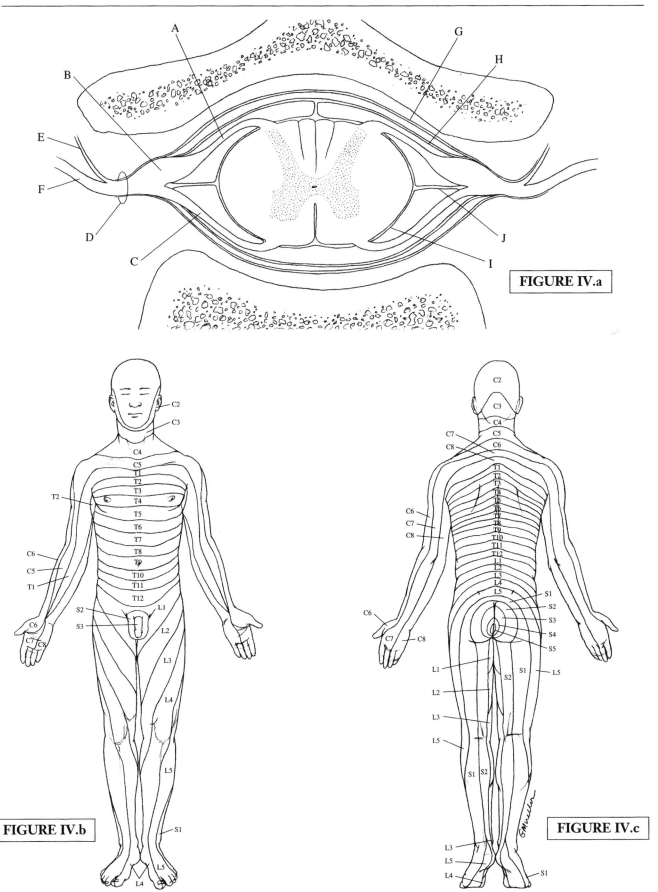

FIGURE IV.a

FIGURE IV.b

FIGURE IV.c

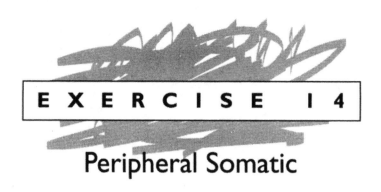

EXERCISE 14

Peripheral Somatic

CERVICAL PLEXUS

This plexus is derived from ventral rami of cervical levels 1-4 (FIGURE 14.1). This plexus lies deep to the internal jugular vein and sternocleidomastoid muscle. A distinguishing feature is the *ansa cervicalis* (A), a nerve loop from C_1 to C_3. The superior root hitches a ride with the hypoglossal nerve before joining with the branches of the inferior root. The nerves of this plexus supply the skin and muscles of the neck as well as the thoracic diaphragm. Its components and their functions are:

Lesser occipital nerve (B), sensory to the skin of the neck and posterior scalp.
Great auricular nerve (C), sensory to the area around the parotid gland and ear.
Transverse cervical nerve (D), sensory to the anterior neck.
Supraclavicular nerves (E) arise as one trunk splits into three branches to supply the skin in the area of the clavicle.

These nerves all make their superficial appearance in the mid-lateral neck between the posterior border of the sternocleidomastoid muscle and the anterior border of the trapezius muscle. This area is sometimes described as the punctum nervosum.

A small portion of the superior root of the ansa sends a motor branch to the thyrohyoid muscle and branches from the loop innervate the infrahyoid muscles: omohyoid, sternothyroid, and sternohyoid.

The *phrenic nerve* (F), arises primarily from C_4, with some contribution from C_3 and C_5. It descends on the anterior surface of the anterior scalene muscle. This is the only motor nerve of the plexus and supplies the thoracic diaphragm. It enters the thorax via the superior thoracic aperture anterior to the subclavian artery and is often found adherent to the pericardium.

❓ FOR REVIEW AND THOUGHT

Cervical vertebral dislocation above C_3 is catastrophic and very often fatal. Why?

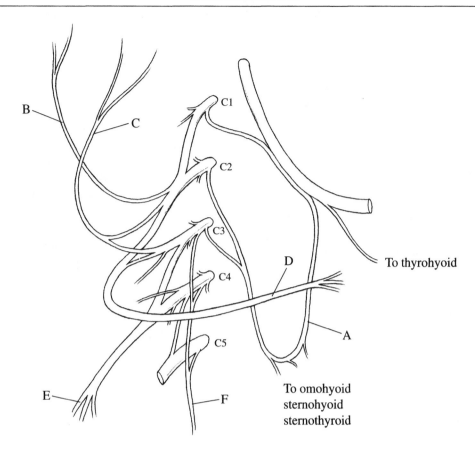

C1

C2

C3

D

C4

To thyrohyoid

A

C5

To omohyoid
sternohyoid
sternothyroid

B

C

E

F

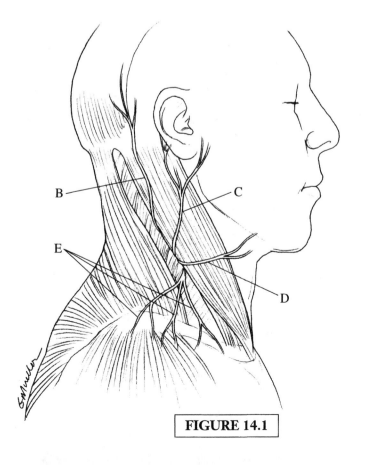

B

C

E

D

FIGURE 14.1

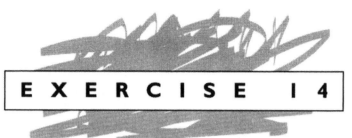

Peripheral Somatic

BRACHIAL PLEXUS

This plexus is found in the region commonly known as the armpit. The anatomical name for this region is the *axilla*: an area of extreme importance, containing not only this plexus but the major arterial and venous vessels of the upper limb. (The familiar shoulder wound of westerns, war movies, and detective dramas is no minor matter; but rather a devastating, and possibly fatal wound.) The brachial plexus is structurally and functionally well organized. A key to understanding this plexus is the '**M**' identified by the probe in FIGURE 14.2. Deep to the probe are two major nerves (axillary and radial) which supply the posterior surface of the limb, and lifted by the probe are the three major nerves to the anterior surface (musculocutaneous, median, and ulnar). Let's begin our study!

Origin

Ventral primary rami from cervical nerves 5-8 and thoracic nerve 1 (C_5-T_1).

Roots

Join to form *trunks* (color red).
1. superior trunk, from $C_{5,6}$
2. middle trunk, from C_7
3. inferior trunk, from C_8, T_1

Trunks

Join to form *divisions* (color orange).
4. anterior divisions – nerves from these are destined to supply anterior (flexor) muscles
5. posterior divisions – nerves from these are destined to supply posterior (extensor) muscles

Divisions

Join to form *cords* (color brown).
6. lateral cord – formed by anterior divisions of the superior and middle trunks
7. medial cord – formed by the anterior division of the inferior trunk
8. posterior cord – formed by the posterior divisions of all three trunks

Cords

Give off *terminal branches*.

From the Lateral Cord
9. musculocutaneous nerve – motor to anterior arm muscles (color violet)
10a. 1/2 of the median nerve (color green)

From the Medial Cord
10b. 1/2 of the median nerve – motor to most of the anterior forearm muscles, the thenar muscles, and the lateral two lumbricals (color blue) (color the united median nerve blue-green) (10)
11. ulnar nerve – motor innervation to 1 1/2 muscles of the anterior forearm, the intrinsic muscles of the hand and the medial two lumbricals (color red-orange)

From the Posterior Cord
12. axillary nerve – motor to the deltoid and teres minor (color yellow)
13. radial nerve – motor to the posterior muscles of the arm and forearm (color light brown)

Collateral Branches

From roots, trunks, and cords, but not from divisions (color as per their site of origin: root, red; trunk, orange, etc.)

From Roots
14. dorsal scapular nerve – from C_5; motor to the rhomboids and the levator scapulae
15. long thoracic nerve – from C_{5-7}; motor to the serratus anterior

From Trunks
16. suprascapular nerve – from the superior trunk; motor to the supraspinatus and infraspinatus
17. nerve to the subclavius – from the superior trunk; motor to the subclavius

From the Lateral Cord
18. lateral pectoral nerve – motor to the pectoralis major

From the Medial Cord
19. medial pectoral nerve – motor to the pectoralis major and minor
20. medial brachial cutaneous – sensory to the medial surface of the arm
21. medial antebrachial cutaneous – sensory to the medial surface of the forearm

From the Posterior Cord
22. upper subscapular nerve; motor to the subscapularis
23. thoracodorsal nerve – motor to the latissimus dorsi
24. lower subscapular nerve – motor to the subscapularis and teres major

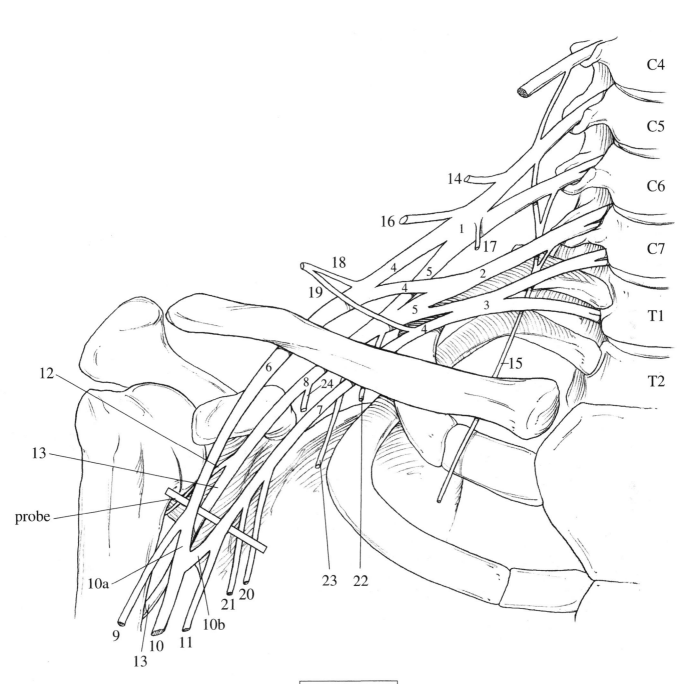

FIGURE 14.2

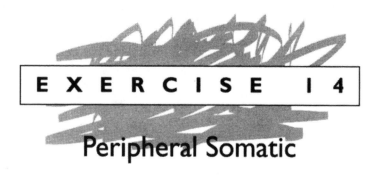

EXERCISE 14

Peripheral Somatic

The five major nerves of the upper limb: musculocutaneous, axillary, radial, ulnar, and median are mixed and also carry sensory neurons to their areas of muscular distribution. This sensory distribution is shown in FIGURE 14.3.

MUSCULOCUTANEOUS NERVE

After supplying the muscles of the anterior arm, it yields the lateral cutaneous nerve of the arm and the lateral cutaneous nerve of the forearm.

MEDIAN NERVE

The nerve is named for its course (right down the middle of the upper limb). It is sensory to the thumb, second and third phalanges and half of the fourth phalanx.

ULNAR NERVE

As you well know this nerve becomes quite superficial as it reaches the elbow and passes directly posterior to the medial epicondyle of the humerus. It has no branches in the arm. It is also sensory to the palmar surface of digit five and medial half digit four.

AXILLARY NERVE

This nerve wraps around the posterior aspect of the surgical neck of the humerus accompanied by the posterior humeral circumflex vessels. Because of this position, it is vulnerable to damage in mid-shaft fractures of the humerus. Note its sensory distribution!

At, or slightly inferior to the elbow, the nerve splits into superficial and deep branches. The superficial branch will yield five dorsal digital nerves that are sensory to the posterior surface of the thumb and the lateral two fingers.

RADIAL NERVE

After wrapping around the shaft of the humerus, the radial nerve continues into the forearm. It provides sensory innervation to the posterior arm and forearm and continues to the hand where it branches to supply the posterior surface of the thumb and adjoining two and a half fingers.

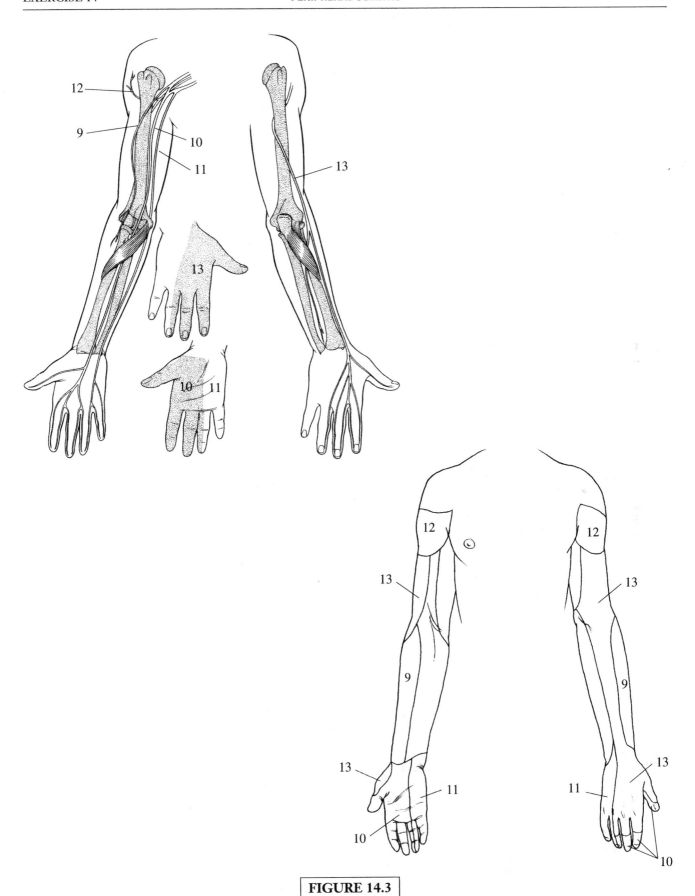

FIGURE 14.3

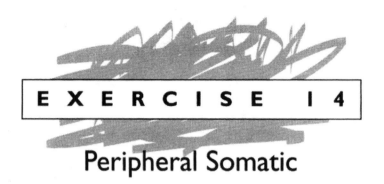

EXERCISE 14

Peripheral Somatic

LUMBOSACRAL PLEXUS

This plexus (FIGURE 14.4) is formed by ventral primary rami of lumbar and sacral nerves. Branches from L_{1-3} form the lumbar portion, with its roots within the psoas major muscle. The sacral portion arises from $L_{4,5}$ and S_{1-4}. Like the brachial plexus anterior and posterior divisions are present, which join to form nerves. Because of the medial rotation of the lower limb during embryonic development, nerves formed by posterior divisions come to supply anteriorly placed muscles and nerves formed by anterior divisions come to supply posteriorly placed muscles. The basic concept of posterior nerves supplying extensors and anterior nerves supplying flexors still holds, however.

LUMBAR PLEXUS

Nerves from Anterior Divisions

1. Ilioinguinal nerve (L_1) – sensory to the external genitalia; motor to the abdominal wall
2. Genitofemoral nerve ($L_{1,2}$) – divides into genital and femoral branches; the genital branch travels with the spermatic cord into the scrotum (or with the ligamentum teres into the labia major in the female); supplies the cremaster muscle, and is sensory to the skin of the external genitalia and medial thigh; the femoral branch is sensory to the thigh in the region of the femoral triangle
3. Obturator nerve (L_{2-4}) – motor to the muscles of the adductor (medial) compartment of the thigh (color blue)

Nerves from Posterior Divisions

4. Iliohypogastric nerve (L_1) – supplies the skin of the gluteal region via a lateral branch and the skin over the inguinal ligament via an anterior branch
5. Lateral femoral cutaneous ($L_{2,3}$) – sensory to the lateral thigh
6. Femoral nerve (L_{2-4}) – motor to the iliacus, psoas major, psoas minor, and the muscles of the anterior thigh (color sky blue). The remainder of L_4 and all of L_5 join to form the lumbosacral trunk, connecting the lumbar and sacral plexuses

SACRAL PLEXUS

Nerves from Anterior Divisions

7. Tibial nerve (L_5, S_{1-3}) – motor to most of the posterior thigh, posterior leg, and plantar surface of the foot (color red)
8. Pudendal nerve (S_{2-4}) – sensory to the genitalia; motor to perineal muscles and sphincter urethrae, external anal sphincter and levator ani
9. Nerve to the superior gemellus and obturator internus (L_5, $S_{1,2}$)
10. Nerve to the quadratus femoris and inferior gemellus ($L_{4,5}$, S_1)

Nerves from Posterior Divisions

11. Common peroneal nerve ($L_{4,5}$, $S_{1,2}$) motor to the short head of the biceps femoris; muscles of the lateral leg, anterior leg, and dorsum of the foot via superficial and deep peroneal branches (color orange)
12. Superior gluteal nerve ($L_{4,5}$, S_1) – motor to the gluteus medius and minimus, and the tensor fascia latae (color green)
13. Inferior gluteal nerve (L_5, $S_{1,2}$) – motor to the gluteus maximus (color yellow-green)
14. Nerve to the piriformis ($S_{1,2}$) (color yellow)
15. Posterior femoral cutaneous nerve (S_{1-3}). This nerve is formed by posterior divisions of $S_{1,2}$ and anterior divisions of $S_{2,3}$

The tibial and common peroneal nerves are usually united within a connective tissue sheath to form the *sciatic nerve* (A) (color red-orange). This is most clearly seen in the deep gluteal region. These nerves will separate in the inferior thigh.

❓ FOR REVIEW AND THOUGHT

Review the passage of the sciatic nerve through the gluteal region. Might this be endangered in gluteal injections? Where should such injections be administered?

Compare the structure, organization, and distribution of the nerves of the brachial and lumbosacral plexuses. What is similar? What is different? Why?

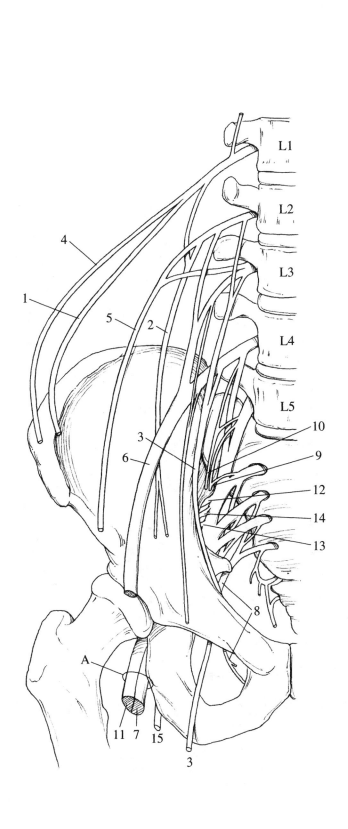

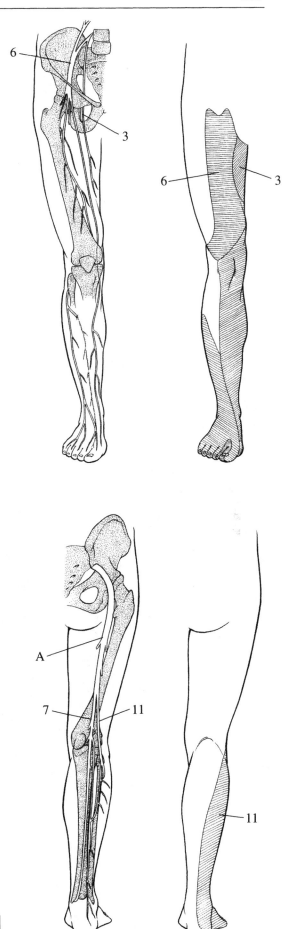

FIGURE 14.4

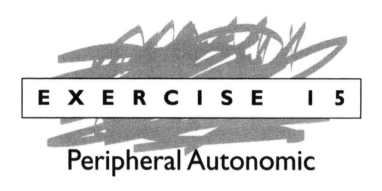

EXERCISE 15

Peripheral Autonomic

The autonomic nervous system provides motor innervation to smooth muscle, cardiac muscle, and glands. The route traversed to target structures is quite different from that of somatic nerves. The nerves we have just finished studying passed from the ventral horn of the spinal cord to their targets along only one neuron.

Autonomic nerves have their cell bodies in the lateral horn of the spinal cord and require two neurons in their functional pathway (FIGURE 15.1). A *preganglionic neuron* (A) (color yellow) passes from its origin in the lateral horn and synapses with the *cell body of the postganglionic neuron* (B) in a ganglion located outside the central nervous system. (Thus the designation as peripheral.) The activation of the postganglionic neuron produces the effect of this system. In fact the postganglionic neuron (color orange) is called the "effector."

The autonomic portion of the peripheral nervous system is subdivided into two differing, yet complementary, portions: sympathetic and parasympathetic. The cell bodies of the preganglionic neurons of the sympathetic portion are found in the thoracic and lumbar regions of the spinal cord, while those of the parasympathetic are located in cranial nerves and the sacral region of the cord. The sympathetic portion tends to have relatively short preganglionic and relatively long postganglionic neurons; with the parasympathetic showing just the opposite: long preganglionic and short postganglionic. Finally the effector chemical for postganglionic neurons differs: epinephrine for sympathetic and acetylcholine for parasympathetic.

Generally these two systems work in contradiction or opposition to maintain involuntary processes for function of the individual and continuation of the species. Heart rate, oxygen content in the blood, digestion, adjustment of the lenses of the eye for near/distant vision, and erection and ejaculation, are just some examples of their work. Let's make one statement as a reference point for your learning: *the sympathetic portion is excitatory and the parasympathetic is regulatory (calming)!* This is not exactly true but it does serve as a guide.

SYMPATHETIC (THORACOLUMBAR)

The preganglionic cell bodies of this portion of the autonomic nervous system originate in the thoracic and lumbar regions of the spinal cord (T_1-L_2). Associated closely is the *sympathetic trunk* (C), a chain of connected ganglia along both sides of the vertebral column from cervical to coccygeal levels (FIGURE 15.1). Sympathetic preganglionic neurons leave the spinal cord and enter the ganglion via *white rami communicantes* (D). Once in the ganglion these neurons may ascend or descend in the ganglionic chain, pass through to other specifically named ganglia, or synapse with a postganglionic neuron which then exits the ganglion via a *gray rami communicans* (E) (color gray) to join a spinal nerve. No matter the particular route two things are consistent: the system works via two neurons and ganglia are quite distant from the organs innervated; resulting in relatively long postganglionic neurons.

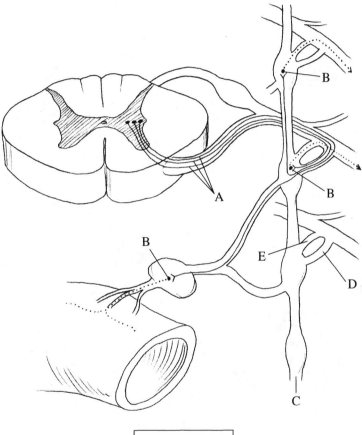

FIGURE 15.1

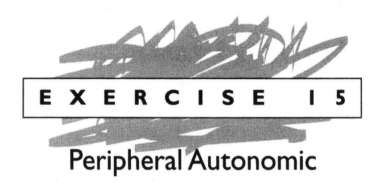

EXERCISE 15

Peripheral Autonomic

PARASYMPATHETIC (CRANIOSACRAL)

The parasympathetic portion of the autonomic nervous system has cell bodies in the brain stem and in the lateral horn of the spinal cord: level S_{2-4}. Four parasympathetic ganglia are found in the head (FIGURE 15.2).

The *ciliary ganglion* (F) is found in the orbit, just lateral to the optic nerve. Short postganglionic neurons pass to the eyeball as short ciliary nerves to innervate the sphincter and ciliary muscles for accommodation of the pupil.

The *pterygopalatine ganglion* (G) is suspended from the maxillary nerve in the pterygopalatine fossa. Post ganglionic fibers pass to the lacrimal and nasal glands as well as the mucus membrane and glands of the nose, throat, and palate: producing secretion.

The *otic ganglion* (H) is located inferior to the foramen ovale on the medial side of the mandibular division of the trigeminal nerve. From this ganglion postganglionic fibers pass to the parotid gland to produce secretion.

The *submandibular ganglion* (I) receives preganglionic fibers from the facial nerve. Postganglionic fibers pass to the sublingual and submandibular glands: producing secretion.

The sacral parasympathetic nerves leave the spinal cord as preganglionic neurons and unite as the *pelvic splanchnic nerves* (J) (FIGURE 15.3). The preganglionic neurons synapse at ganglia near, or within the walls of, the organs they innervate and the very short postganglionic neurons are the effectors. Stimulation of the pelvic splanchnics produces voiding of the bladder, dilatation of blood vessels, and penile (or clitoral) erection.

❓ FOR REVIEW AND THOUGHT

Identify sympathetic and parasympathetic influences on the following organs or processes:

heart
    duodenum
    respiration
    adrenal hormones

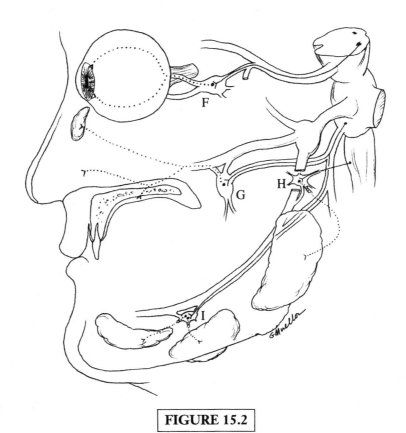

FIGURE 15.2

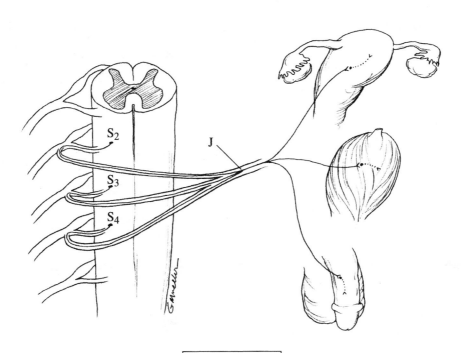

FIGURE 15.3

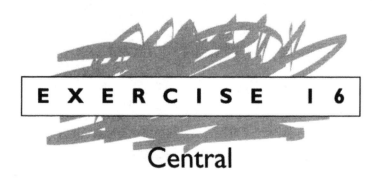

EXERCISE 16

Central

SPINAL CORD

The spinal cord extends from the foramen magnum to the level of the first or second lumbar vertebra (FIGURE 16.1) and shows *cervical* (A) and *lumbar (B)* enlargements indicating the levels of the nerves to and from the limbs. The cord presents an *anterior median fissure* (C) and a *posterior median sulcus* (D). Dorsal and ventral rootlets of spinal nerves attach lateral to these midline features.

Three neural plexuses (L., braid; a network or tangle) (FIGURE 16.1) arise from the spinal cord: *cervical* (C_1-C_4), supplying the lateral and anterior neck; *brachial* (C_5-T_1), supplying the upper limb; and *lumbosacral* (L_1-S_4), supplying the gluteal region, pelvis, and lower limb. These plexuses are composed of ventral primary rami of spinal nerves. While these, especially the brachial and lumbosacral, may seem incredibly complex they do possess a certain degree of organization.

The lumbosacral plexus is particularly instructive in terms of the relationship between the spinal cord and the vertebral column. In the adult the cord is shorter than the vertebral column and some nerves are dragged inferiorly to reach their appropriate level of exit from the vertebral column. These nerves gather in what is called the *cauda equina* (E), from its resemblance to a horse's tail. The cord terminates as the *conus medullaris* (F) which continues as a fine thread, the *filum terminale* (G), an anchoring structure destined to attach to the dorsum of the coccyx.

❓ FOR REVIEW AND THOUGHT

Discuss with a study partner the significance of the region you have just studied. Be able to answer the following questions.

1. What processes brought about the formation of the cauda equina and surrounding subarachnoid space?
2. What is the significance of this region for diagnostic and anesthetic purposes?

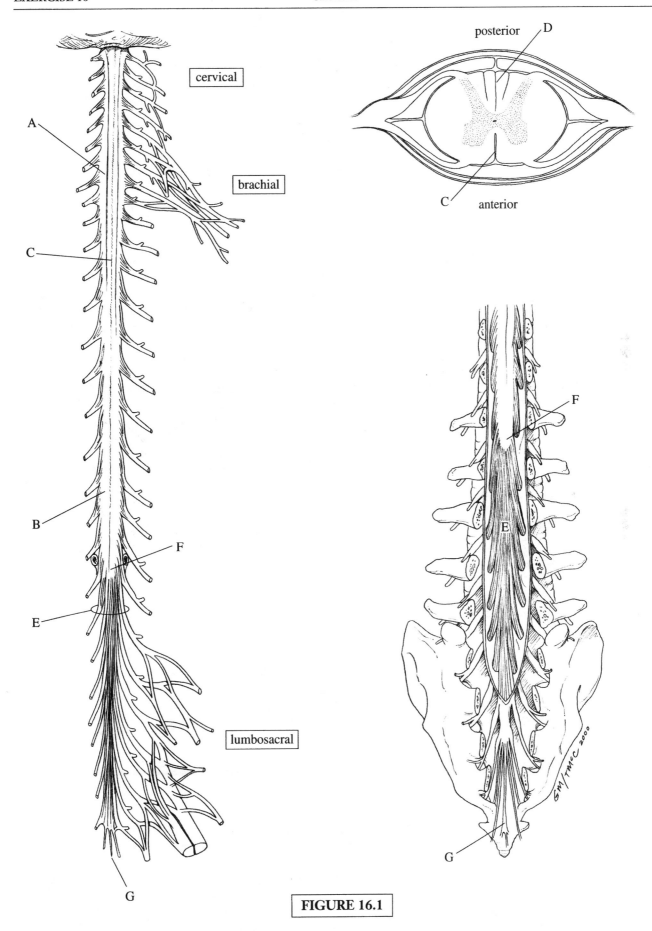

FIGURE 16.1

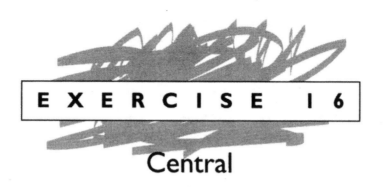

Central

BRAIN

The intent here is not to provide an exhaustive account of brain structure and function but to relate these to sensory and motor needs of the human. The paired cerebral hemispheres account for the largest portion of the brain (FIGURE 16.2a and FIGURE 16.2b). Each is divided into four lobes: *frontal* (color bar: yellow), *parietal* (color bar: orange), *temporal* (color bar: red-orange), and *occipital* (color bar: red).

The surface of the hemispheres is characterized by *sulci* (grooves) and *gyri* (elevations). By this folding the surface area of the brain is greatly increased. Two thirds of all the surface area of the cortex is found in the depths of the sulci. Two prominent sulci are the *central* (A) and *sagittal* (B). The sagittal separates the two hemispheres of the brain. The central sulcus plays a more important role, separating the frontal lobes from the parietal lobes, but more importantly the *precentral gyrus* (C) of the frontal lobes (with the motor cortex) from the *postcentral gyrus* (D) of the parietal lobes (with the general sensory cortex).

The cerebrum shows a *lateral sulcus* (E) separating the temporal lobe from the frontal and parietal lobes. This sulcus is quite deep and involves the overlapping of a deep portion of cerebral cortex, the *insula* (F), by portions of the parietal and temporal hemispheres: the *opercula* (H).

A midline view (FIGURE 16.2c) shows the *corpus callosum* (I), composed of commissural fibers passing between cerebral hemispheres; bounded by the *cingulate gyrus* (J). The area inferior to the corpus callosum is the *midbrain* (color yellow-green): featuring the *thalamus* (K) and *hypothalamus* (L), the *pituitary gland* (M) seated in the *sella turcica* (N), and the *pineal gland* (O). The remainder of the brainstem includes the *pons* (color green) and *medulla oblongata* (color sky blue). Inferior to the occipital lobes, and tucked under a transverse fold of dura mater, the *tentorium cerebelli* (P), are the paired lobes of the *cerebellum* (color violet).

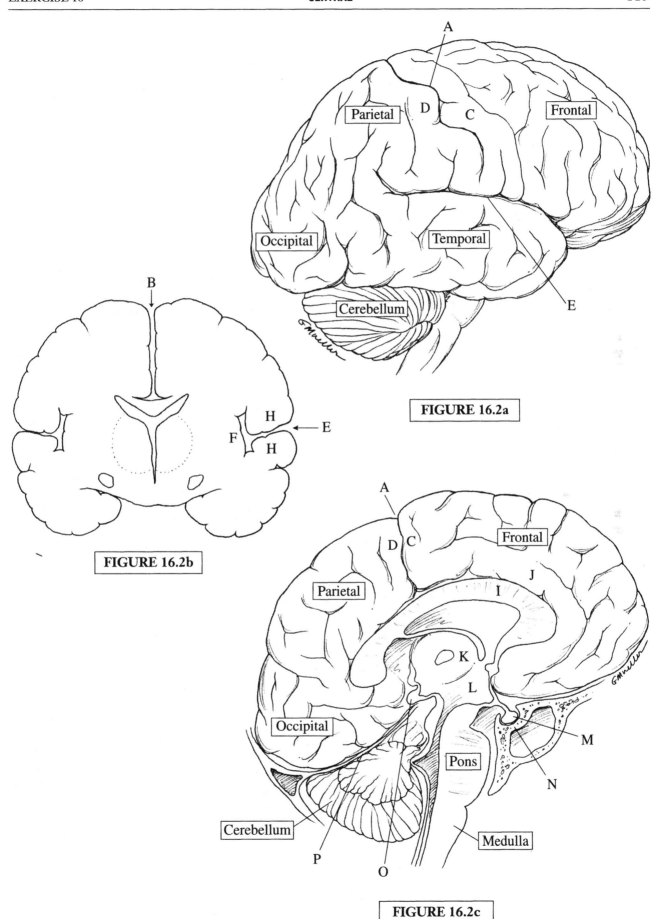

FIGURE 16.2a

FIGURE 16.2b

FIGURE 16.2c

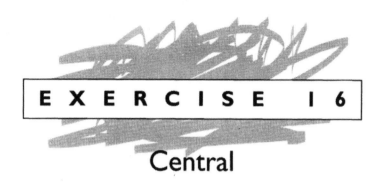

EXERCISE 16

Central

BRAIN (CONTINUED)

As is the case with the entire central nervous system the brain is surrounded by the three meningeal layers (dura, arachnoid, and pia maters) with cerebrospinal fluid in the arachnoid layer. In addition a series of ventricles and channels are found in the brain for the production and passage of cerebrospinal fluid (FIGURE 16.3a).

Each cerebral hemisphere has a large *lateral ventricle* (Q) with *anterior* (Q_1), *central* (Q_2), *inferior* (Q_3), and *posterior* (Q_4) *horns.* The lateral ventricles have extensive tufts of vascular villi, *choroid plexus* (R), that secrete cerebrospinal fluid. In the anterior horn of each lateral ventricle is a small channel, the *interventricular foramen of Monro* (S), leading to the midline *third ventricle* (T). The roof of the third ventricle also has choroid plexus (FIGURE 16.3b, c).

From the third ventricle cerebrospinal fluid passes into the *fourth ventricle* (U) via the *cerebral aqueduct of Sylvius* (V). Once again the roof of this ventricle includes choroid plexus.

Cerebrospinal fluid flows from the lateral ventricles, through the third ventricle, and into the fourth ventricle. In the fourth ventricle it escapes into the subarachnoid space of the central nervous system via three channels. A midline posterior *foramen of Magendie* (W), and bilateral *foramina of Luschka* (X). A continuation of the cerebral aqueduct remains as the central canal of the spinal cord (Y).

❓ FOR REVIEW AND THOUGHT

What is the function (purpose) of cerebrospinal fluid?

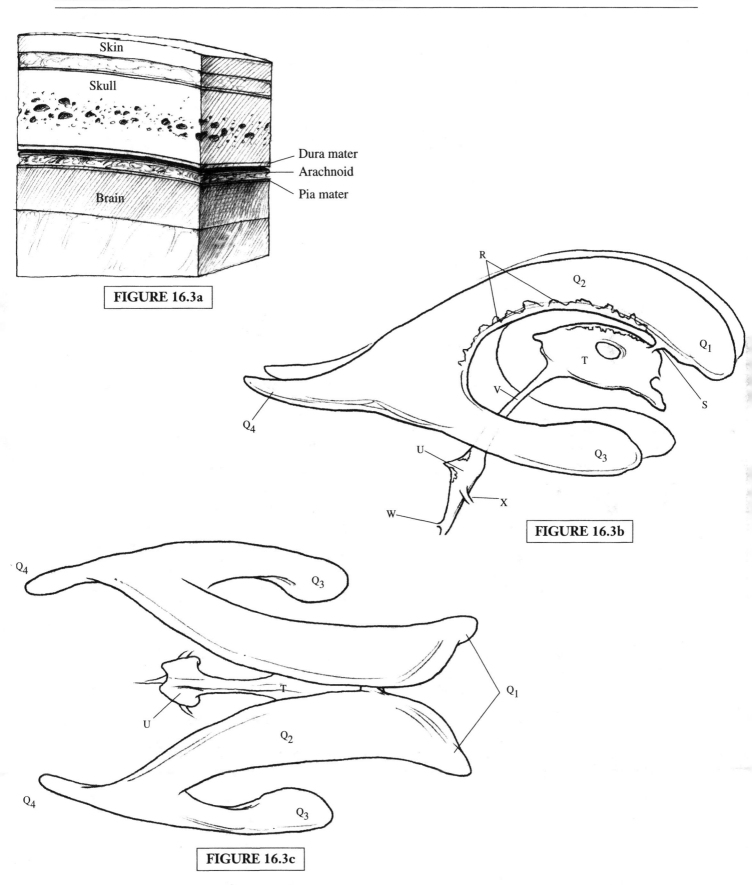

FIGURE 16.3a

FIGURE 16.3b

FIGURE 16.3c

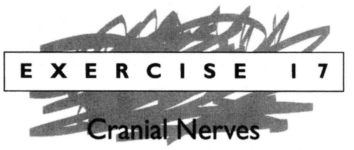

Cranial Nerves

A detailed description and study of the cranial nerves is fascinating and difficult. In our work we will attempt to describe the anatomic relationships and functional significance of these special nerves. Use FIGURE 17.1a to aid in your conceptualization of these nerves, their pathway, and their function. Use the table to enter your notes in each cell. Included within the table is the foramen of exit of each nerve. This is of importance in understanding the course a nerve or branch takes (see pages 122–123).

Cranial nerves have their origin from the brain or brainstem and may be composed of as many as four different types of neurons: special sensory, general sensory, motor, and autonomic (parasympathetic). Most are not; possessing only one or two types of neurons (FIGURE 17.1b, c).

CRANIAL NERVE I: OLFACTORY

Carries **special sensory** fibers for smell. This nerve is actually attached to the underside of the telencephalon; the most primitive sensory area of the brain. The sense of smell is the oldest of all senses. Olfactory neurons hanging through the foramina of the cribriform plates of the ethmoid bone congregate as *olfactory bulbs* (A) and transmit to the brain via the *olfactory tracts* (B).

CRANIAL NERVE II: OPTIC

Carries the **special sense** of sight. The fibers carrying this sense arise from the ganglion cells of the retina. From the retina it passes through the optic canal to enter the cranium. The *optic nerves* (C) meet and partially cross at the *optic chiasma* (D).

CRANIAL NERVE III: OCULOMOTOR

This is a mixed nerve carrying **motor** (no surprise given its name) and **parasympathetic preganglionic** neurons. It has its origin in the midbrain. The motor neurons innervate four of the six extraocular muscles: *inferior oblique* (E), *medial* (F), *superior* (G) and *inferior rectus* (H), and the *levator palpebrae superioris* (I). The preganglionic parasympathetic neurons are destined to synapse in the *ciliary ganglion* (J). Postganglionic neurons pass to the involuntary muscles that constrict the eye and change the shape of the lens (accommodation).

CRANIAL NERVE IV: TROCHLEAR

This slender nerve arises from the midbrain and is purely **motor** supplying only one extraocular eye muscle: the *superior oblique* (K). It takes its name from the fact the superior oblique muscle passes through pulley (L., trochlea) in its course to a distal attachment on the eyeball.

CRANIAL NERVE VI: ABDUCENS (F)

Question: What happened to Cranial Nerve V?.
Answer: *It is so interesting, complicated, and fun that it needs its own page. We'll get to it soon!*

The abducens nerve derives its name from the one extraocular muscle it innervates: the *lateral rectus* (L) (an abductor of the eyeball). The origin of this **motor** nerve is in the pons.

CRANIAL NERVE VIII: VESTIBULOCOCHLEAR

Yes, another nerve has been skipped: Cranial Nerve VII. It, too, is interesting and complex and has several functional and physical interactions with V, so be patient.

The vestibulocochlear nerve (M) originates in separate portions of the inner ear, and is truly two nerves travelling together. The vestibular portion is responsible for proprioceptive information from the maculae of the saccule and utricle and the ampullae of the semicircular canals. The cochlear nerve carries impulses from the Organ of Corti in the cochlea: the **special sense** of hearing.

CRANIAL NERVE IX: GLOSSOPHARYNGEAL

Although it is primarily sensory this nerve includes all four possible types of neurons. The tongue and pharynx are its areas of distribution: thus its name. **Motor** fibers innervate the *stylopharyngeus muscle* (N). General **sensory** fibers innervate the posterior third of the tongue, the wall of the pharynx, and the middle ear. **Special sensory** fibers convey taste from the posterior third of the tongue. **Parasympathetic preganglionic** fibers pass to the *otic ganglion* (O).

CRANIAL NERVE XI: SPINAL ACCESSORY

Wait! We skipped another nerve! Yes, the vagus nerve has wandered onto another page also.

The cranial portion of this **motor** nerve arises from the medulla and is destined to join the vagus nerve, supplying the muscles of the soft palate and the intrinsic muscles of the larynx. The spinal root ascends from C_{5-1}, exits the jugular foramen in company with the cranial portion, and passes to the *sternocleidomastoid* (P) and *trapezius* (Q) muscles, which it innervates.

CRANIAL NERVE XII: HYPOGLOSSAL

This **motor** nerve exits the skull via the hypoglossal canal. It innervates the intrinsic and extrinsic muscles of the tongue.

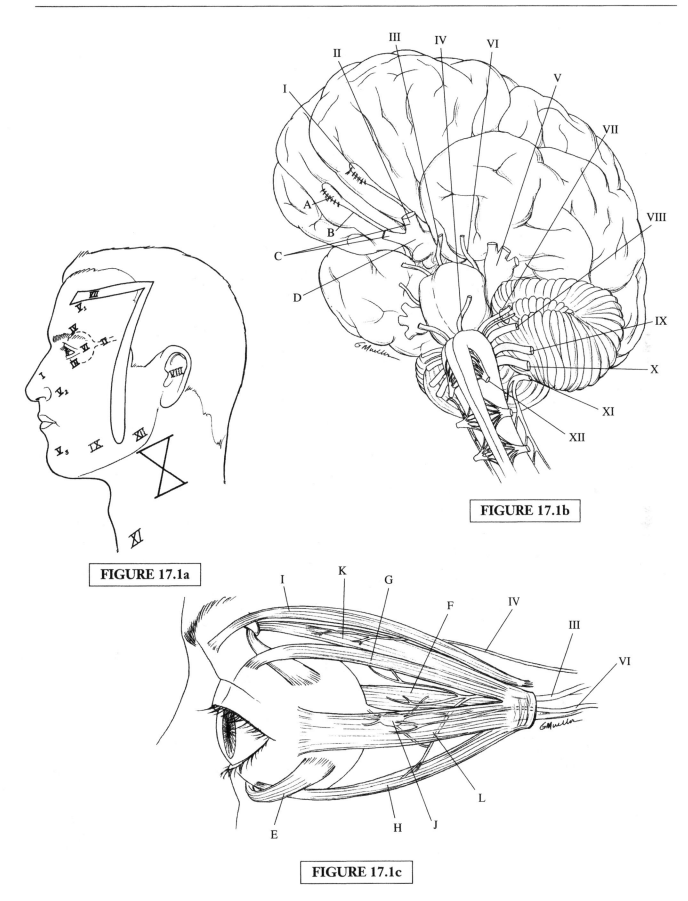

FIGURE 17.1a

FIGURE 17.1b

FIGURE 17.1c

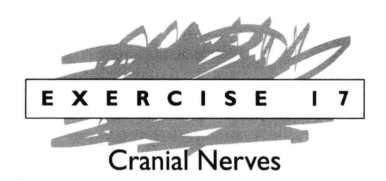

EXERCISE 17

Cranial Nerves

The trigeminal, facial, and vagus nerves are worthy of enhanced scrutiny because of their great variety of functions and destinations.

CRANIAL NERVE V: TRIGEMINAL

The branches of this nerve (FIGURES 17.2 and 17.3) carry general **sensory** neurons for the head and **motor** neurons for the muscles of mastication. A general description of the distribution of this nerve is: a superior branch to the forehead and scalp, a middle branch to the maxillae, and an inferior branch to the mandible and mouth. The inferior branch is mixed: sensory and motor. This nerve has a physical, but not functional, relationship with all four parasympathetic ganglia.

V_1 OPHTHALMIC (COLOR YELLOW)

This nerve enters the orbit through the superior orbital fissure. Within the orbit several important branches arise.

A. Frontal nerve
    1. supratrochlear – medial corner of the eye
    2. supraorbital – conjunctiva, skin of the upper eyelid, and the scalp as far posterior as the vertex
B. Lacrimal nerve – lacrimal gland
C. Nasociliary nerve
    4. branch to the ciliary ganglion
    5. long ciliary nerves – eyeball
    6. infratrochlear – skin of the nose

V_2 MAXILLARY (COLOR ORANGE)

The maxillary nerve leaves the skull through the foramen rotundum and passes beneath the floor of the orbit to its exit onto the face via the infraorbital foramen.

D. Zygomatic nerve – temporal region, skin over the zygomatic arch
E. Pterygopalatine nerve – superior pharynx, nasal cavity, hard and soft palates
F. Infraorbital nerve – skin between the lower eyelid and the upper lip

V_3 MANDIBULAR (COLOR RED-ORANGE)

After its passage through the foramen ovale it gives off three sensory branches. It also gives off motor branches to the muscles of mastication.

G. Auriculotemporal nerve – skin of the temporal region, external auditory meatus, and tympanic membrane
H. Lingual nerve – general sense to the anterior two thirds of the tongue
I. Inferior alveolar nerve – sensory innervation to the lower teeth and gums. Also motor supply to the mylohyoid and anterior belly of the digastric.
    7. mental – skin of the tip of the chin

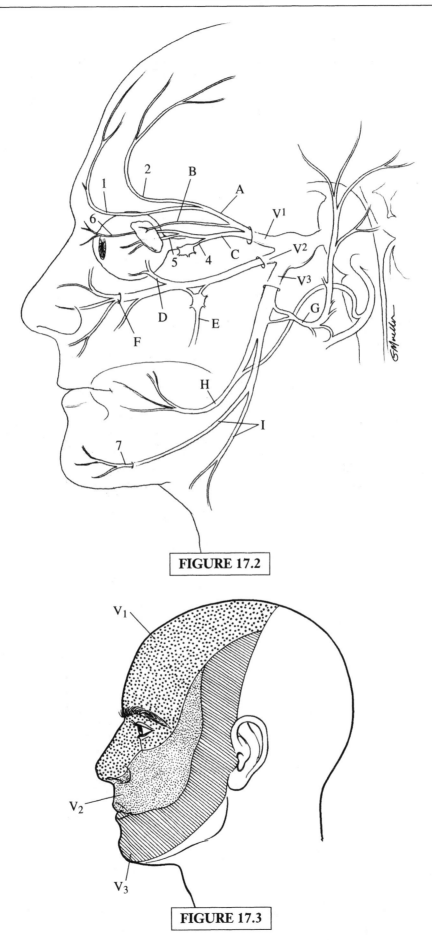

FIGURE 17.2

FIGURE 17.3

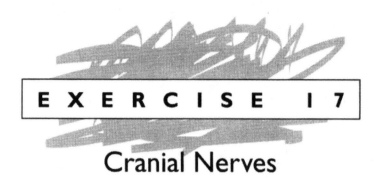

EXERCISE 17

Cranial Nerves

CRANIAL NERVE VII: FACIAL (COLOR GREEN)

The facial nerve (FIGURE 17.4) is primarily **motor** to the muscles of facial expression. The nerve exits the skull through the stylomastoid foramen, passes deep to the parotid gland, and sends five branches to the face.

J. Temporal
K. Zygomatic
L. Buccal
M. Mandibular
N. Cervical

Parasympathetic preganglionic neurons pass from this nerve to the *pterygopalatine* (O) and *submandibular ganglia* (P). A **sensory** component innervates the tongue, palate, and external ear. **Special sensory** fibers for taste from the anterior two thirds of the tongue are carried in the *chorda tympani* (Q). This nerve 'hitches a ride' from the tongue with the lingual branch of V_3, separates to unite with the main nerve and enters the skull through the stylomastoid foramen.

CRANIAL NERVE X: VAGUS (COLOR SKY BLUE)

The vagus nerve is a wanderer (FIGURE 17.5) . Its name derives from the Latin meaning just that. This nerve arises from the medulla and branches throughout the neck, thorax, and abdomen as far as the distal end of the transverse colon. This nerve is composed primarily of **preganglionic parasympathetic** neurons to affect the carotid sinus, heart, lungs, digestive organs, and associated glands but also contains some of each of the other three types of neurons. **Motor** fibers pass to the muscles of the larynx and pharynx. **Sensory** fibers from the sense organs for pain in the skin of the external auditory meatus and **special sensory** fibers for taste from the area of the epiglottis and stretch receptors in the walls of the great vessels and the lung.

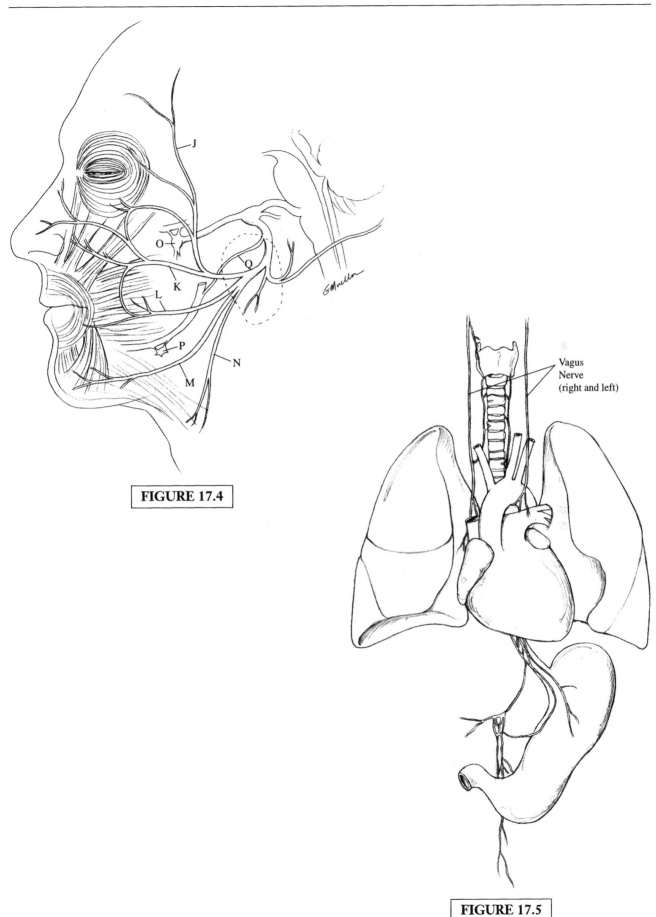

FIGURE 17.4

Vagus
Nerve
(right and left)

FIGURE 17.5

CRANIAL NERVES

NAME	MOTOR	SENSORY	SPECIAL SENSORY	AUTONOMIC	FORAMEN OF EXIT
I					
II					
III					
IV					
	V_1				
	V_2				
	V_3				

VI

VII

VIII

IX

X

XI

XII

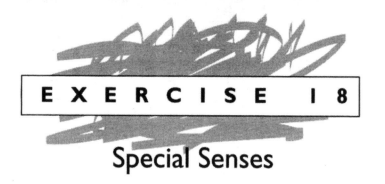

OLFACTION

The sense of smell is phylogenetically the oldest and one might say the most basic of all the senses. In most of the animal kingdom it is instrumental in survival and in stimulating behavior. A decrease in this sense with aging, or the common cold, is a nuisance for humans but certainly not life threatening. As vision is used more exclusively the dependence upon olfaction decreases.

Olfactory neurons are found in the mucosa of the *superior and supreme conchae* (A) (FIGURE 18.1). (Thus the need to sniff to thoroughly enjoy a particularly pleasing odor like chocolate chip cookies in the oven.) From these neurons the sense passes to paired *olfactory bulbs* (B) (color yellow) and *olfactory tracts* (C) (color orange), which will terminate in the rhinencephalic (smell brain) portion of the underside of the forebrain (D). Alone among the senses, olfaction has no primary projection to the thalamus.

VISION

Vision occurs when light from an object strikes the retina. Rods and cones in the retina are sensitive to light and color respectively. It has been estimated these cells compose nearly 70% of all receptors in the body!

Light is sensed on the retina in a prescribed way. The nasal aspect of each retina receives light from the periphery of the visual field and the temporal retina receives light from central sources of the visual field (FIGURE 18.2). From the retina each *optic nerve* (E) courses to the *optic chiasma* (F) where the neurons from the nasal portion of each retina cross. The newly formed *optic tracts* (G) now contain fibers from the temporal portion of their own eye and the nasal portion of the contralateral eye. The tracts pass to, and synapse in, the lateral geniculate nuclei in the thalamus. Axons from the thalamus pass to the striate area of the occipital cortex as *optic radiations* (H).

Accommodation of the lens of the eye is also critical. This process, by which the refractive power of the lens is changed for near or distant vision, involves the cerebral cortex when one decides to focus on distant or near objects. Pupillary constriction/dilatation in response to bright/dim light and dilatation are reflex actions of significance as well (FIGURE 18.3).

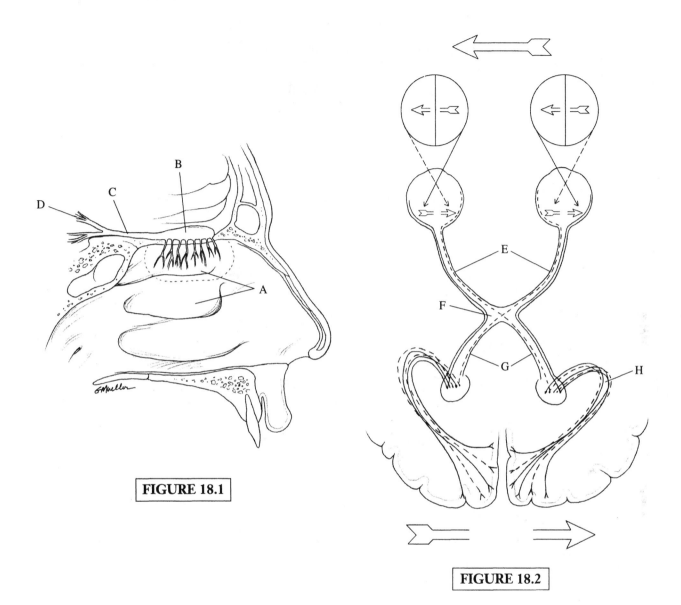

FIGURE 18.1

FIGURE 18.2

Constriction   Dilatation

FIGURE 18.3

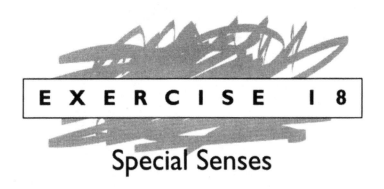

EXERCISE 18

Special Senses

TASTE

Cranial Nerves VIII, IX, and X carry taste from the *taste buds* (A) of the tongue and epiglottis (FIGURE 18.4). A close association of taste and smell makes our discussion a bit more complex. The association of taste with flavor also includes memory. This involves evaluation/appreciation of spices, textures of foods, temperature, 'chemical heat' of foods such as jalapeno peppers, or the 'tang' of various cheeses. Even the sight and/or sounds of the creation of various foods may awaken taste buds.

Pure taste, without the influence of smell, is a chemical event and involves only four sensations: sweet, sour, salt, and bitter. These sensations are located in specific areas of the tongue (B): sweet on the tip, salt on the periphery, sour in the middle, and bitter on the back. (Thus the term: leaving a bad taste in your mouth!) A given taste bud responds to no more than one of the four classical tastes. Taste impulses pass to the ventral posteromedial nucleus of the thalamus and thence to the inferior aspect of the postcentral gyrus.

AUDITION

Hearing is associated with a portion of Cranial Nerve VIII and the membranous labyrinth of the inner ear; including the semicircular canals, the utricle and saccule associated with the vestibular system, and the cochlear duct for audition.

Audition begins with vibrations impacting on the tympanic membrane, the boundary between the outer and middle ear (FIGURE 18.5a). The three tiny bones of the middle ear: *malleus* (C), *incus* (D), and *stapes* (E), transfer, convert, or enhance these vibrations. Two tiny muscles: tensor tympani and stapedius (see page 92) are involved in dampening or magnifying these vibrations. Large amplitude/low volume vibrations at the eardrum are converted to low amplitude/large force vibrations at the *oval window* (F).

The *cochlear duct* (G) (FIGURE 18.5b and 18.5c) contains the *Organ of Corti* (H) coursing its entire length in 2¾ loops and composed of two parallel tubes: the *scala vestibuli* (I) and *scala tympani* (J). These vibrations are converted into pressure waves within the fluid (perilymph) of the inner ear. *Hair cells* (K) acting as mechanoreceptors transduce the wave into a neural impulse that passes in the cochlear portion of Cranial Nerve VIII to the medial geniculate nuclei in the thalamus. Axons from the thalamus pass to the temporal gyrus of Heschl in the cerebral cortex.

❓ FOR REVIEW AND THOUGHT

What is the final destination of all these senses?

Once you have answered this does the phrase "In your mind's eye!" take on new significance?

Think of, and list, the associations you have made between special senses and memory! Here are some to help you: chocolate chip cookies, new pajamas, and mom's pot roast.

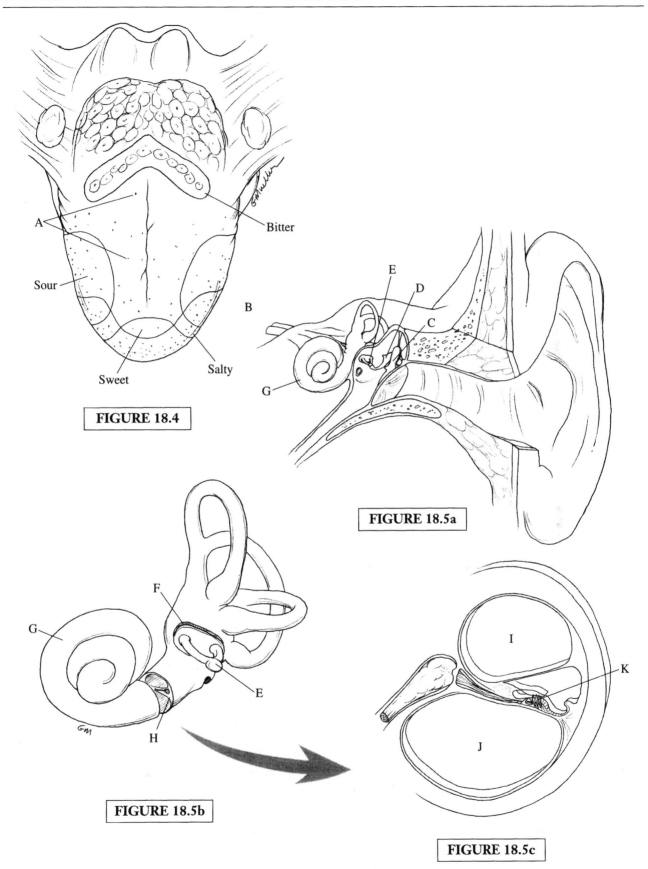

FIGURE 18.4

FIGURE 18.5a

FIGURE 18.5b

FIGURE 18.5c

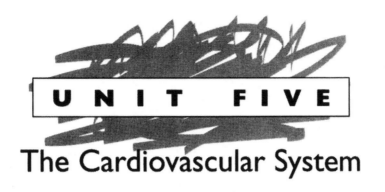

UNIT FIVE

The Cardiovascular System

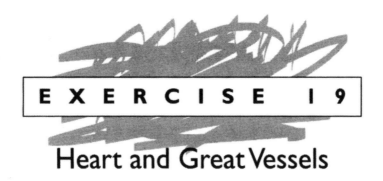

EXERCISE 19

Heart and Great Vessels

The cardiovascular system is structured around a centrally located pumping station (the heart) with outflow valves and piping (arteries) to deliver oxygen-rich blood to working sites (muscles, glands, organs) and a somewhat different type of piping (veins) for return of oxygen-deficient blood. Schematic views of this arrangement are shown in FIGURES 19.1 and 19.2. Also shown is a conceptual representation of the postnatal circulation, with oxygen rich blood depicted in clear vessels and oxygen-deficient blood in dark vessels.

The heart is a four-chambered pump which is postnatally divisible into pulmonary and systemic circuits (FIGURE 19.2). The pulmonary portion (right chambers) pumps oxygen-deficient blood to the lungs while the systemic portion (left chambers) pumps oxygen-enriched blood to the entire body. Keep this premise clearly in mind and both prenatal and postnatal heart function will make sense, as will the changes in circulation occurring at, and shortly after, birth.

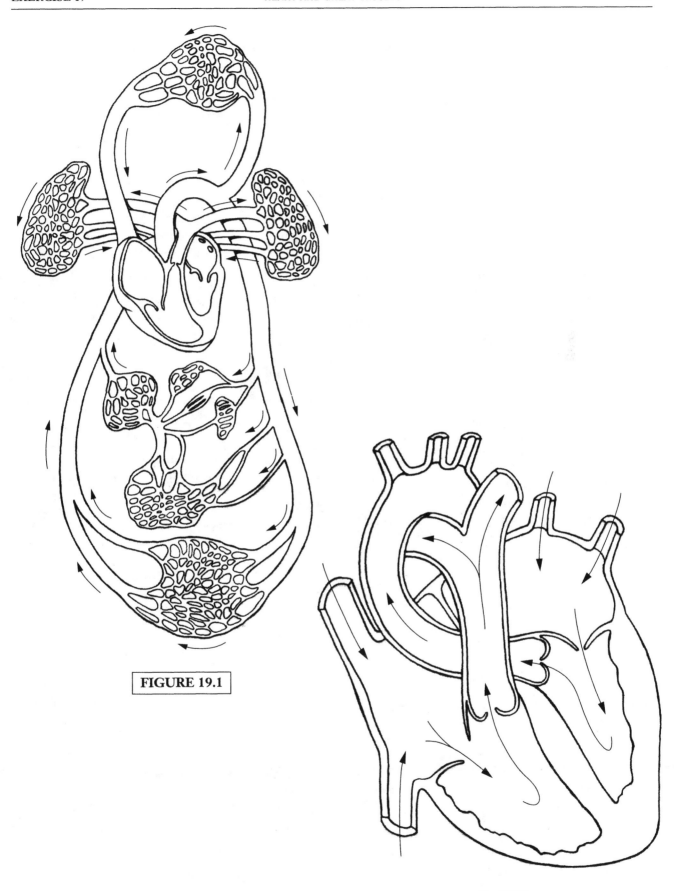

FIGURE 19.1

FIGURE 19.2

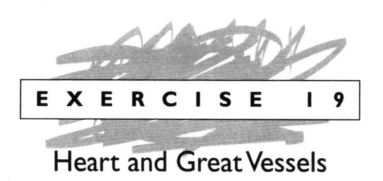

Heart and Great Vessels

Viewed anteriorly, portions of all chambers of the heart are visible as well as the great vessels entering and leaving (FIGURE 19.3). In such a view the surrounding *fibrous pericardium* (A) is seen to follow the great vessels for some distance. A thinner layer, the *visceral pericardium* (B), intimately covers the exterior surface of the heart. Orientation to the chambers of the heart is facilitated by finding the *superior* (C) and *inferior venae cavae* (D) emptying into the right atrium. Once done the *right ventricle* (E) is the main feature in this view. The *pulmonary trunk* (F) and *aortic arch* (G) are also shown.

RIGHT ATRIUM

This chamber (H) receives venous blood from the venae cavae. Externally it shows a prominent *auricle* (H_1), extending anteriorly. A significant internal feature on the medial wall is the *fossa ovalis* (H_2), the remains of the foramen ovale, a prenatal shunt between the atria. Also obvious is the opening of the inferior vena cava with its valve, or lip, which served to direct blood toward the foramen ovale during fetal life. Almost immediately inferior to the fossa is the opening of the *coronary sinus* (H_3), the main venous drainage of the heart.

RIGHT VENTRICLE

The opening into this ventricle (I) is characterized by an atrioventricular valve (the *tricuspid valve* [I_1]) with three cusps: *anterior* (I_2), *posterior* (I_3) and *medial* (I_4) papillary muscles are connected to the cusps via *chordae tendineae* (I_5). During right ventricular contraction the papillary muscles also contract, tensing the chordae tendineae and preventing reversal of the cusps into the right atrium.

The exit from the right ventricle via the pulmonary trunk features a different form of valve. The *pulmonary semilunar valve* (I_6) prevents backflow of blood into the right ventricle during ventricular filling. This valve is composed of three cusps which flop toward one another, meeting in the center of the trunk during ventricular filling and pushed against the wall of the trunk during ventricular contraction and the ejection of blood. The free edge of each cusp shows a slight thickening, the *nodule* (I_7) on its free edge. The three nodules meet centrally, forming a seal to prevent backflow (FIGURE 19.4).

LEFT ATRIUM

This rather unremarkable chamber (P) could reasonably be called the posterior atrium, since it 'hides' behind the left ventricle. Oxygen-rich blood from the lungs enters this chamber via four *pulmonary veins* (P_1) (only the left veins are shown). The orifice between this and the ventricle features a *bicuspid valve*. (Routinely called the *mitral valve* due to its fancied resemblance to a bishop's mitre.)

LEFT VENTRICLE

The opening into the *left ventricle* (Q) is via the *bicuspid (mitral) valve* (Q_1). It has the same function as does the tricuspid and is also equipped with papillary muscles and chordae tendineae to each cusp: *anterior* (Q_2) *and posterior* (Q_3) (FIGURE 19.5). Their task is considerably more daunting, however, due to the much greater pressure exerted during left ventricular contraction. Note the anterior cusp of the valve has surfaced facing both the inflow of blood from the atrium and the outflow of blood from the ventricle. For this reason, this cusp is sometimes called the "aortic cusp."

The cavities of both ventricles, but especially the left, show many *trabeculae carneae* (R): muscular ridges covering much of the interior walls. Note that the two ventricles share a common wall: the *interventricular septum* (S).

The aortic semilunar valve is stationed at the base of the aorta. Like the pulmonary valve each cusp has a nodule on its free surface aiding the cusps in joining to form a seal. The right and left coronary arteries arise from the right and left *aortic sinuses* (T): cups formed between the free lips of the cusps and the wall of the aorta.

Functionally, the Aortic Semilunar Valve Is a Masterpiece!

Closure of the valve during left ventricular filling is assisted by retrograde accumulation of the last portion of blood just ejected from the ventricle. Opening of the semilunar valve during the next ventricular contraction assists in pushing pooled blood in these sinuses into the coronary arteries.

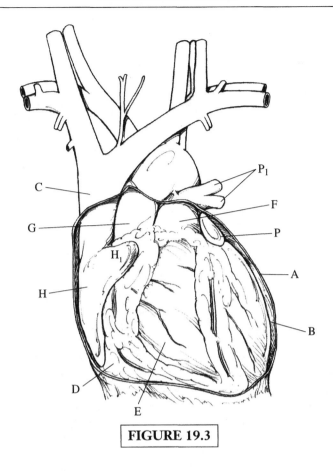

FIGURE 19.3

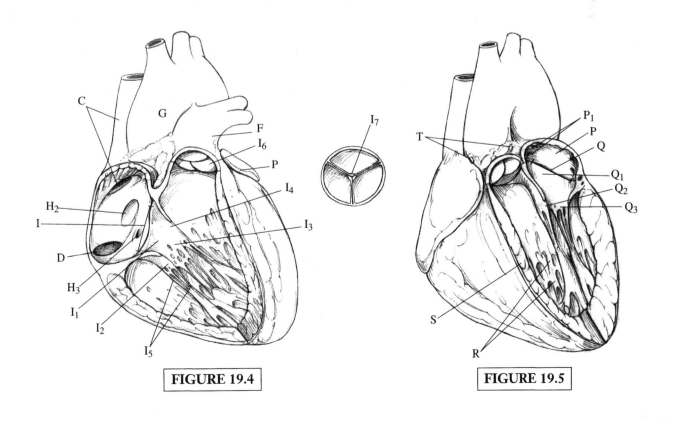

FIGURE 19.4   **FIGURE 19.5**

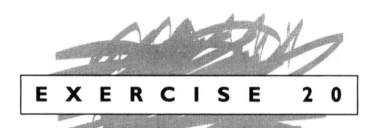

EXERCISE 20

Arterial Supply and Venous Drainage of the Heart

As the aorta leaves the left ventricle its first two branches are encountered: the *right* (A) and *left* (B) *coronary arteries.* (FIGURES 20.1 and 20.2) These two vessels and their branches will supply oxygen-rich blood to the four chambers of the heart. Most commonly the left coronary artery splits to form *anterior interventricular* (C) (sometimes called descending) and *circumflex* (D) branches. The anterior interventricular artery lies in the anterior interventricular sulcus and courses toward the apex of the heart. It is destined to continue this path, pass to the posterior surface of the heart, and ascend in the posterior interventricular sulcus before anastomosing with the *posterior interventricular* (E) branch of the right coronary artery. The circumflex artery courses in the coronary sulcus between the left atrium and ventricle to reach the posterior surface of the heart where it *anastomoses* (F) with the termination of the right coronary artery. The coronary arteries are often obscured by fat. The same is true of the coronary sinus, the main venous drainage of the heart.

The right coronary artery descends in the coronary sulcus between the right atrium and ventricle. Its first major branch is the *marginal artery* (G) that passes along the inferior margin of the heart toward the apex. The right coronary artery continues around the posterior side of the heart to give off the posterior interventricular artery before anastomosing with the circumflex branch of the left coronary. All of these arteries send their branches into the depth of the heart musculature.

The *great cardiac vein* (H) is found accompanying the anterior interventricular artery and will become the *coronary sinus* (I). The *posterior vein of the left ventricle* (J) runs from the left margin of the heart to empty into the great cardiac vein or the coronary sinus. The *middle cardiac vein* (K) runs with the posterior interventricular artery and empties into the coronary sinus, which in turn empties into the right atrium. *Anterior cardiac veins* (L), draining the right atrium and ventricle, typically empty into the right atrium independent from the coronary sinus.

❷ FOR REVIEW AND THOUGHT

What is the anatomy of a heart attack?

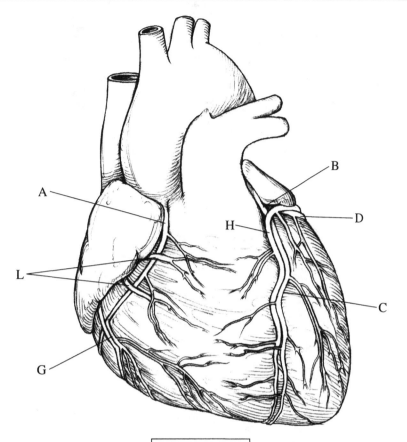

FIGURE 20.1

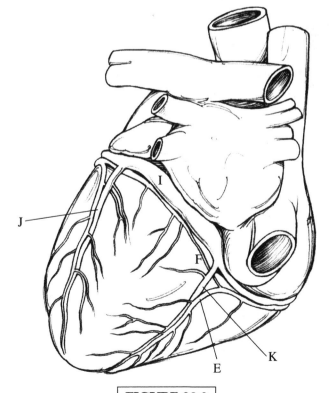

FIGURE 20.2

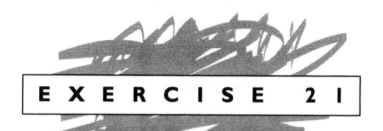

EXERCISE 21

Arterial Supply and Venous Drainage of the Neck and Head

As the aorta ends its ascent and begins to arch toward its inferior path three major branches are found (FIGURE 21.1). The first is the *brachiocephalic trunk* (A), destined to supply the right upper limb (brachium) via the *subclavian artery* (B) and the right side of the neck and head (cephalo) via the *common carotid artery* (C). (On the left side of the arch the common carotid and subclavian arteries arise separately.) Beginning with the common carotids the arterial supply is 'the same' on each side of the neck and head. The common carotid arteries are destined to split into *internal* (D) and *external* (E) branches at approximately the level of the superior border of the thyroid cartilage. The carotid sinus and carotid body are located at this bifurcation.

EXTERNAL CAROTID ARTERY

Ascends to supply the exterior of the neck, face, and head. Eight major branches are usually described.

F. Superior thyroid – thyroid gland
    1. superior laryngeal
G. Ascending pharyngeal – pharynx, palate, tonsils, auditory tube

H. Lingual – tongue; also sends branches to the tonsils, soft palate, and suprahyoid muscles
I. Facial – muscles and skin of face
    2. inferior labial – lower lip
    3. superior labial – upper lip
    4. angular – terminal continuation of the facial; to the medial angle of the eye
J. Occipital – posterior scalp, sternocleidomastoid, trapezius
K. Posterior auricular – external ear and part of the tympanic membrane
L. Maxillary – both jaws, nasal cavity, oral cavity, tympanic membrane, dura mater, lacrimal gland, and eye muscles
    5. inferior alveolar – mandible and lower teeth
    6. middle meningeal – dura mater
    7. buccal – cheek and gums (gingiva)
    8. infraorbital – upper jaw and teeth
    9. sphenopalatine – nasal cavity
M. Superficial temporal

This artery terminates as *frontal* (N) and *temporal* (O) branches.

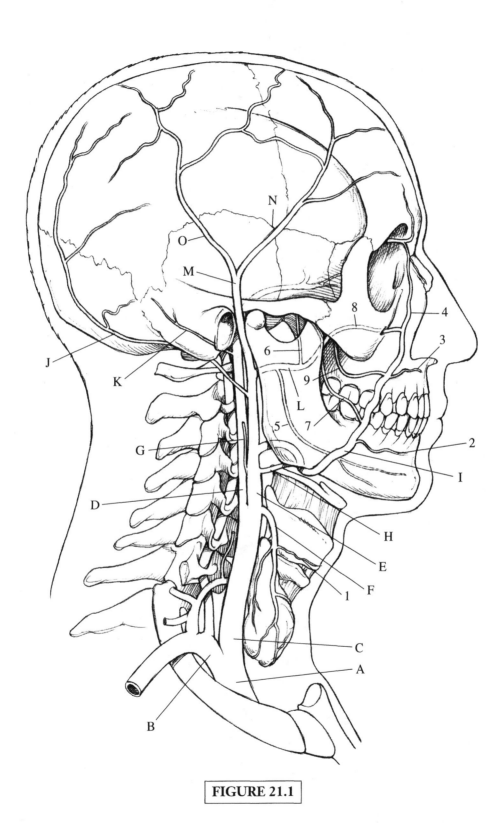

FIGURE 21.1

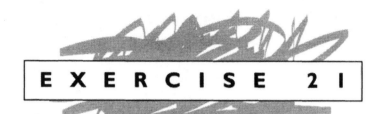

EXERCISE 21

Arterial Supply and Venous Drainage of the Neck and Head

INTERNAL CAROTID ARTERY

This artery has no branches in the neck. It enters the temporal bone and passes through the carotid canal to reach the middle cranial fossa. Once inside the cranium it is a major supplier to the brain. These paired arteries can be found alongside the sella turcica as the legs of the 'rider'. The following branches are usually described (FIGURES 21.2 and 21.3a, b).

A. Ophthalmic – enters the orbit by way of the optic canal
    1. Central artery of the retina
B. Anterior cerebral
    2. Anterior communicating
C. Posterior communicating

D. Anterior choroidal – internal capsule
E. Middle cerebral

The middle cerebral artery is considered the terminal continuation of the internal carotid artery. It and the anterior cerebral will participate in an anastomosis with the vertebral artery: **the Circle of Willis!**

🕐 JUST FOR FUN

With a partner to assist you trace blood from the left ventricle to the right masseter muscle.

Now you assist your partner in tracing blood from the left ventricle to the tympanic membrane!

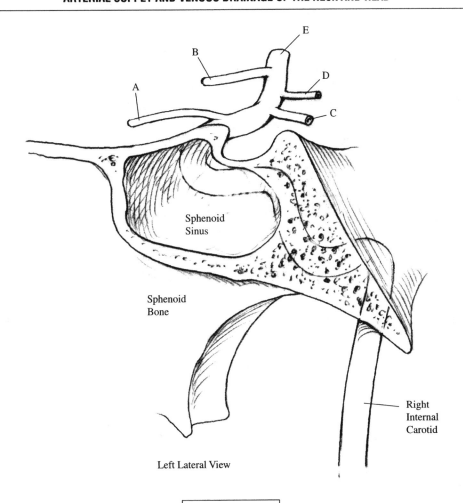

Sphenoid Sinus

Sphenoid Bone

Right Internal Carotid

Left Lateral View

FIGURE 21.2

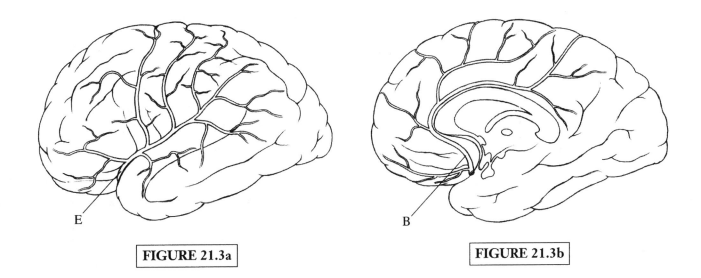

FIGURE 21.3a

FIGURE 21.3b

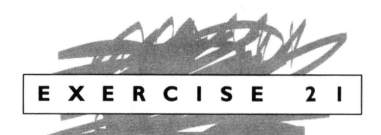

Arterial Supply and Venous Drainage of the Neck and Head

VERTEBRAL ARTERY

The *vertebral arteries* (A) (FIGURE 21.4a) are the first and largest branches off the subclavian arteries. They ascend to the head via the transverse foramina of the cervical vertebrae. After emerging from the transverse foramina of the first cervical vertebra (atlas), they pass dorsally and medially around the superior articular facets and enter the skull through the foramen magnum.

B. Posterior spinal – posterior surface of the spinal cord (paired)
C. Anterior spinal – anterior surface of the spinal cord; paired vessels join to course in the anterior spinal fissure
D. Posterior inferior cerebellar – cerebellum
E. Basilar – formed by the union of the two vertebral arteries
   1. Anterior inferior cerebellar – cerebellum
   2. Labyrinthine – internal ear
   3. Pontine – usually several pairs; supplies pons
   4. Superior cerebellar – cerebellum
   5. Posterior cerebral – terminal branches of the basilar
     a. Posterior communicating

THYROCERVICAL TRUNK

The *thyrocervical trunk* (F) (FIGURE 21.5) is also a branch of the subclavian artery, and supplies blood to neck structures.

G. Inferior thyroid – neck, trachea, esophagus, thyroid gland
   6. Ascending cervical
H. Suprascapular
I. Transverse cervical

CIRCLE OF WILLIS

This is an anastomosis (a communication between two vessels via collateral channels) of the internal carotid and vertebral arteries at the base of the brain, surrounding the pituitary gland and the sella turcica. It is established in the following way: the posterior communicating arteries connect the posterior cerebral arteries with the internal carotid arteries, and the anterior communicating artery connects the two anterior cerebral arteries (FIGURE 21.4b).

❓ FOR REVIEW AND THOUGHT

Arterial supply to the Circle of Willis may take two varying paths. You and your study partner each describe one!

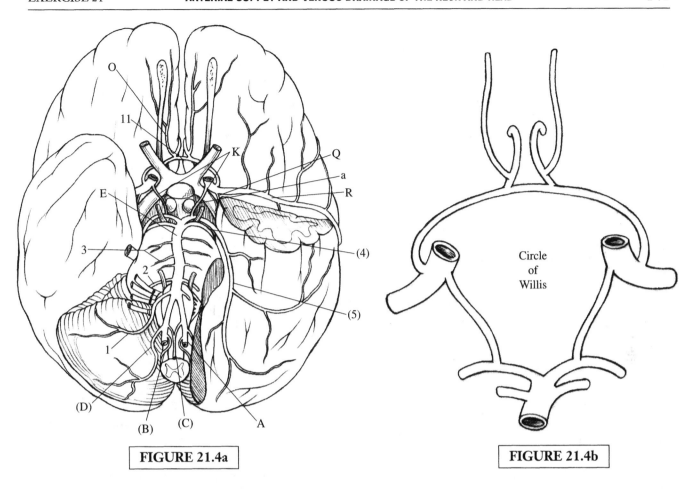

FIGURE 21.4a

FIGURE 21.4b

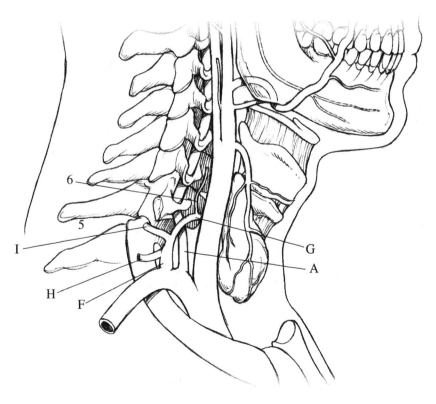

FIGURE 21.5

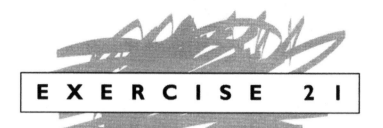

Arterial Supply and Venous Drainage
of the Neck and Head

Venous drainage of the interior of the skull begins in the venous sinuses enclosed within the dura mater (FIGURE 21.6 and 21.7). These sinuses have extensive and quite effective anastomoses with the deep veins of the brain. The *inferior sagittal sinus* (A) flows into the *straight sinus* (B) which, in turn, meets the *superior sagittal sinus* (C). This union is the *confluence of sinuses* (D). From the confluence paired *transverse sinuses* (E) drain laterally. Each makes a sharp 'S-shaped' bend as the *sigmoid sinuses* (F). At the jugular foramina these become the *internal jugular veins* (G). The superior sagittal sinus possesses tufts of *arachnoid granulations* (H). It is here that cerebrospinal fluid produced in the ventricles of the brain diffuses into the sinus for removal via the venous system.

INTERNAL JUGULAR VEIN

The internal jugular vein descends from the jugular foramen within the carotid sheath (in company with the carotid artery and the vagus nerve) and receives venous drainage from superficial areas of the head and neck (FIGURE 21.7). Veins draining into the internal jugular include the following.

I. Facial
J. Anterior branch of the retromandibular
K. Superior thyroid

The internal jugular vein ends by joining the subclavian vein to form the brachiocephalic vein, which continues into the superior vena cava.

EXTERNAL JUGULAR VEIN

The *external jugular vein* (L) receives the greater part of the venous drainage from the exterior surface of the cranium and deep face. It is formed on the external surface of the sternocleidomastoid muscle at about the level of the angle of the mandible by the union of a portion of the retromandibular vein and the posterior auricular vein. It ends by emptying into the subclavian vein. Veins draining into the external jugular include the following.

M. Occipital
N. Posterior auricular

O. Posterior ramus of the retromandibular
　　1. superficial temporal
　　2. maxillary
P. Anterior jugular

Variable in occurrence; typically begins by the union of small veins between the hyoid bone and anterior mandible. It descends near the cervical midline to drain into the external jugular vein near the subclavian vein.

OTHER VEINS

Q. Vertebral

Found in the succeeding transverse foramina of the cervical region; usually as a plexus.

CONNECTIONS BETWEEN SUPERFICIAL AND DEEP VENOUS DRAINAGE

In studying FIGURE 21.7, notice the sites at which these drainages connect. The facial vein connects with the ophthalmic veins in the orbit, and through them with the *cavernous sinus* (R). The facial vein also connects with the *pterygoid plexus* (S) located posterior to the upper molar teeth in the region of the pterygoid plates of the sphenoid bone. The pterygoid plexus, in turn, communicates with the cavernous sinus and, via intercavernous sinuses, the contralateral cavernous sinus. Note the relationship of the *superior* (T) and *inferior petrosal sinuses* (U) with the cavernous sinus. These anastomoses are of considerable clinical importance because the veins of the face are valveless. Infection may pass from superficial to deep veins with potentially devastating results.

❓ FOR REVIEW AND THOUGHT

Return to **JUST FOR FUN** in Exercise 5 (page 34). Does the imagery of the pony express rider make more sense now? All we have to add is the rider, which will be the hypophysis. The cavernous sinuses are the saddle bags and the intercavernous sinuses the straps holding the bags across the saddle!

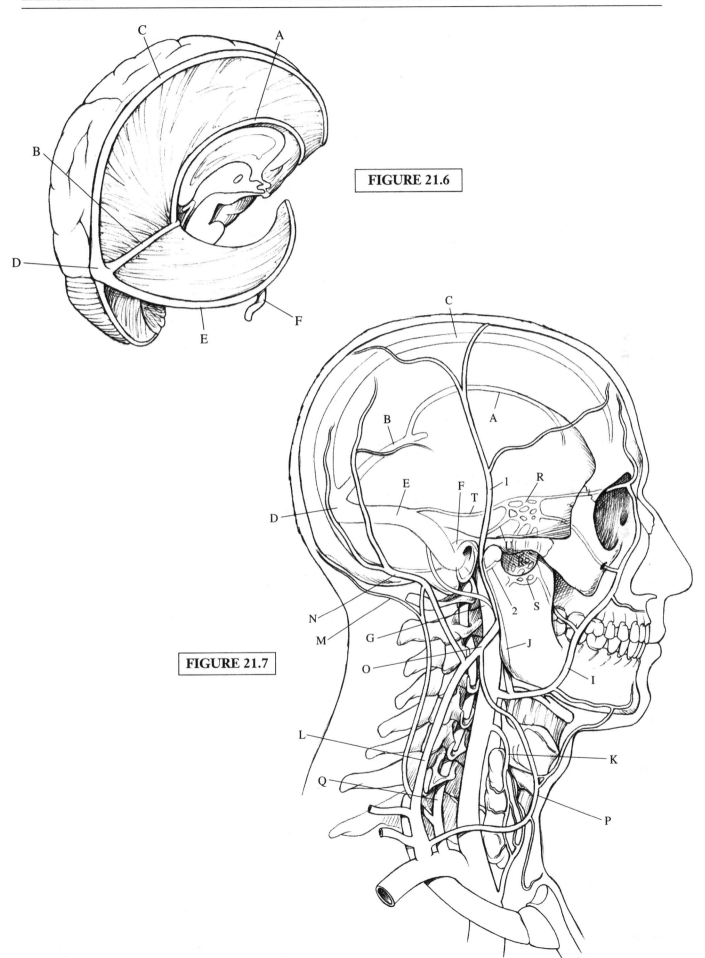

FIGURE 21.6

FIGURE 21.7

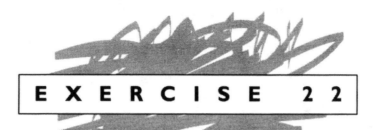

Arterial Supply and Venous Drainage of the Upper Limb

BRACHIOCEPHALIC TRUNK (I)

On the right side, the *subclavian artery* (A) begins as a bifurcation off the brachiocephalic trunk (the other branch is the common carotid). On the left side the subclavian artery is a separate branch off the aortic arch. Each continues to the lateral edge of the first rib. In its course this artery is described in three portions: the first is medial to the scalenus anterior muscle, the second posterior to this muscle, and the third lateral to the muscle. The subclavian artery ends at the lateral edge of the first rib (FIGURE 22.1a).

SUBCLAVIAN ARTERY

B. Vertebral
C. Thyrocervical trunk (FIGURE 22.1b)
 1. Inferior thyroid – thyroid gland
 2. Suprascapular – clavicle and superior scapular area; anastomoses with the scapular circumflex artery
 3. Transverse cervical (sometimes called the descending scapular) – trapezius, levator scapulae, rhomboids, supraspinatus, infraspinatus, subscapularis
D. Internal thoracic – descends to pass along the inner surface of the thoracic wall as far as the diaphragm
 4. anterior intercostal arteries – first six intercostal spaces
 5. musculophrenic arteries – intercostal spaces below 7th intercostal space
E. Costocervical trunk – first two intercostal spaces and muscles of the neck
 6. Deep cervical – posterior neck
 7. Superior intercostal

AXILLARY ARTERY

Part One

Lateral border of the first rib to the superior border of the pectoralis minor (color this part and its branches yellow)

F. Supreme thoracic – first and second intercostal spaces, pectoralis major and minor

Part Two

Deep to the pectoralis minor (color this part and its branches blue)

G. Thoracoacromial trunk – superior and lateral thorax and acromial region of the scapula; long head of the triceps, pectoral muscles, and deltoid
 8. Acromial
 9. Clavicular
 10. Deltoid
 11. Pectoral
H. Lateral thoracic – lateral thorax; pectoral muscles, serratus anterior; and subscapularis

Part Three

Inferior border of the pectoralis minor to inferior border of the teres major (color this part and its branches red)

I. Subscapular
 12. Scapular circumflex – infraspinatus, teres major and minor, deltoid, long head of triceps; forms an anastomosis with the suprascapular
 13. Thoracodorsal – lateral thoracic wall, latissimus dorsi, teres major
J. Posterior humeral circumflex – deltoid, glenohumeral joint
K. Anterior humeral circumflex – coracobrachialis, biceps brachii, glenohumeral joint

BRACHIAL ARTERY

A continuation of the axillary from the inferior border of the teres major to the cubital fossa (color the brachial artery green)

L. Deep brachial (profunda brachii)
M. Nutrient arteries of the humerus
N. Muscular branches
O. Superior ulnar collateral
P. Inferior ulnar collateral

The brachial artery and its branches supply all structures of the arm and participate in the anastomotic network around the elbow joint.

❓ FOR REVIEW AND THOUGHT

What artery is occluded when measuring blood pressure?
 The internal thoracic artery ends by becoming the superior epigastric artery, supplying abdominal muscles.

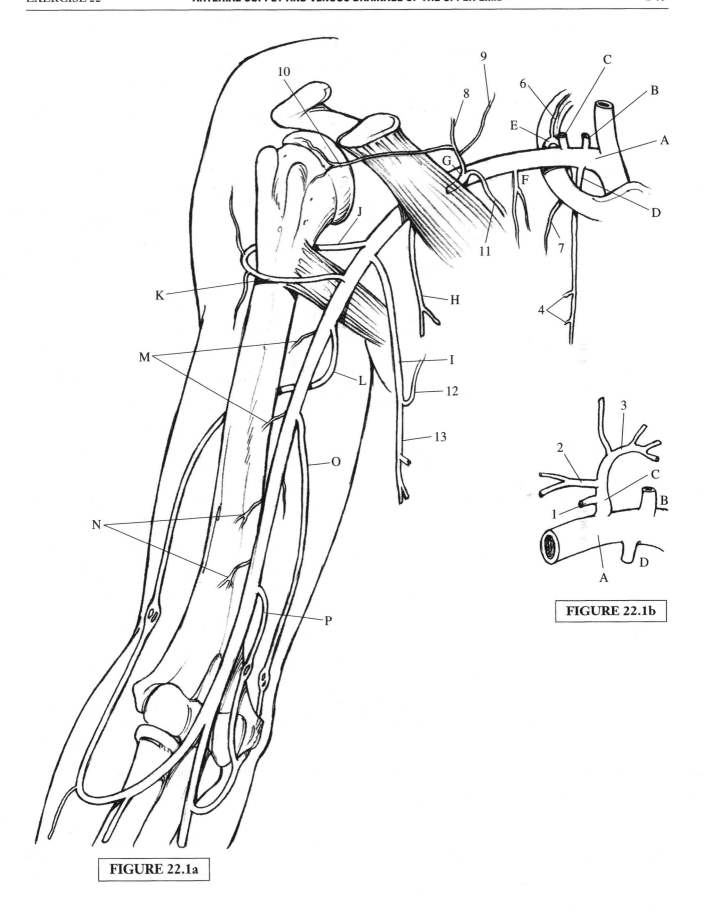

FIGURE 22.1a

FIGURE 22.1b

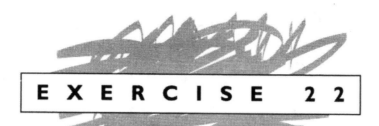

Arterial Supply and Venous Drainage of the Upper Limb

RADIAL ARTERY

As one of the continuing branches of the brachial artery, it courses on the lateral side of the forearm, distributing to structures on this side (FIGURE 22.2a). It supplies most, but not all, of the extensors of the wrist. Branches participate in the anastomosis around the elbow joint and capsule (color this artery and its branches yellow-green).

Q. Radial recurrent
R. Carpal arch – an anastomosis with the ulnar artery
S. Princeps pollicis – main supply to the thumb

ULNAR ARTERY

The ulnar artery bifurcates from the brachial artery at the same point as the radial and continues to the hand, in company with the ulnar nerve. It courses on the medial side of the forearm supplying all structures on this side; including most flexors of the wrist and hand. Branches participate in the anastomosis around the elbow joint and capsule.

Color the ulnar artery and its branches violet.

T. Anterior ulnar recurrent
U. Posterior ulnar recurrent
V. Common interosseous
    12. Anterior – courses on the anterior surface of the interosseous membrane supplying deep structures in the area
    13. Posterior – courses on the posterior surface of the interosseous membrane supplying extensor muscles

SUPERFICIAL AND DEEP PALMAR ARCHES

After giving off the carpal arch the radial and ulnar arteries anastomose to form superficial and deep palmar arches in the hand. These arches, in turn, yield metacarpal and digital branches.

W. Superficial – main supply from the ulnar artery
X. Deep – a continuation of the radial artery

❓ FOR REVIEW AND THOUGHT

What artery is most commonly palpated when taking the pulse?

VENOUS DRAINAGE

The deep veins of the upper limb generally accompany the arteries and are given the same name. Often these accompanying veins (venae comitantes) are paired, and are united by numerous communicating veins. In addition to such deep veins the upper limb also has a superficial set of veins (FIGURE 22.2b).

CEPHALIC VEIN

The *cephalic vein* (A) forms on the dorsum of the hand near the base of the thumb and ascends on the radial side of the limb. In the arm it runs in the lateral bicipital sulcus before reaching the deltopectoral groove through which it passes prior to terminating in the axillary vein.

BASILIC VEIN

The *basilic vein* (B) also begins on the dorsal side of the hand, but ascends along the ulnar side of the forearm. It passes deep at about the midpoint of the arm to join the brachial vein. It continues as the axillary vein at the lower border of the teres major.

The *median cubital vein* (B_1) is a connector between the cephalic and basilic drainage. It usually passes from inferolateral below to superomedial above. It is this vein that is used for venipuncture.

AXILLARY VEIN (C)

This vein is usually described as the continuation of the basilic vein. The deep veins also terminate at about his point and join with the basilic or the first part of the axillary. The axillary vein continues to the first rib, receiving drainage from the cephalic vein and deep veins in the area. At the first rib the axillary continues as the subclavian vein.

SUBCLAVIAN VEIN (D)

This vein receives all the venous blood from the upper limb and joins the internal jugular to form the brachiocephalic vein. The two brachiocephalic veins join to form the superior vena cava.

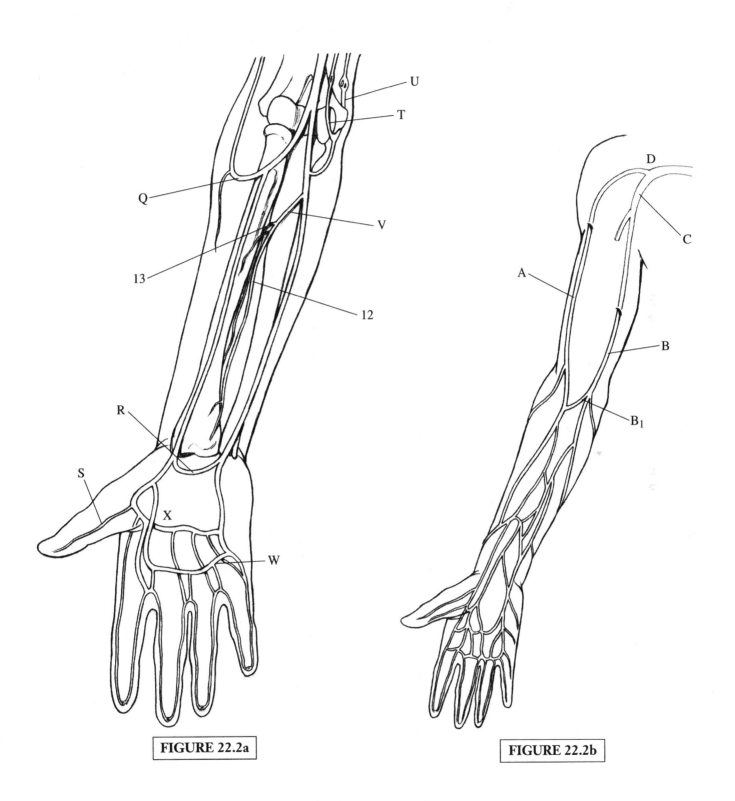

FIGURE 22.2a

FIGURE 22.2b

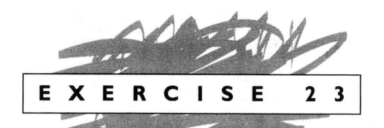

EXERCISE 23

Arterial Supply and Venous Drainage of the Thorax, Abdomen, and Pelvis

Following the branching of the *brachiocephalic trunk* (A), and the left *common carotid* (B), and *subclavian arteries* (C) the aorta descends in the thorax yielding the following branches.

THORACIC AORTA (FROM THE LOWER BORDER OF T$_4$ TO THE DIAPHRAGM) (FIGURE 23.1)

D. Bronchial
E. Esophageal
F. Pericardial
G. Mediastinal

H. Posterior intercostal – usually nine pairs; supply intercostal spaces 3-11
I. Subcostal – inferior to rib 12 (not pictured)
J. Superior phrenic – to posterior surface of the diaphragm

The *internal thoracic artery* (K) also contributes to the arterial supply of the thorax via the following branches.

K$_1$: Anterior intercostal – intercostal 1-6
K$_2$: Musculophrenic – intercostal spaces 7 and below and abdominal muscles
K$_3$: Superior epigastric – the terminal continuation of the internal thoracic; abdominal musculature

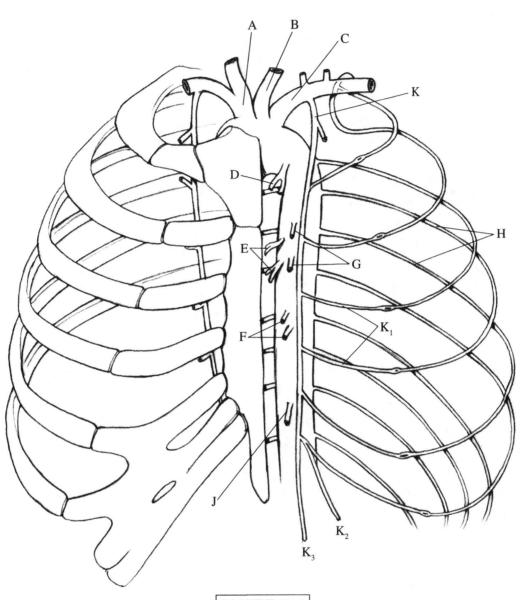

FIGURE 23.1

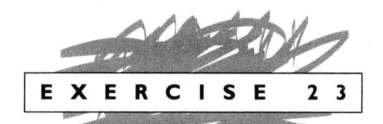

EXERCISE 23

Arterial Supply and Venous Drainage of the Thorax, Abdomen, and Pelvis

ABDOMINAL AORTA (FROM THE DIAPHRAGM TO THE BIFURCATION AT L4 LEVEL)

Several schemes exist for describing the branches of the abdominal aorta. In the present outline the branches are grouped by function and derivation rather than sequential order or origin from the aorta (which is variable from one subject to another in any case).

Letters H-J represent unpaired visceral branches supplying embryonic fore, mid, and hindgut respectively (FIGURE 23.2).

H. Celiac trunk (color yellow)

Arises from the anterior surface of the aorta immediately inferior to the crura of the diaphragm; T_{12} level
1. Left gastric – lesser curve of stomach
2. Common hepatic – liver
   a. Gastroduodenal
      (1) Superior pancreaticoduodenal
      (2) Right gastroepiploic – greater curve of stomach from right to left
   b. Right gastric – lesser curve of stomach from right to left
   c. Proper hepatic – continuation of common hepatic to liver
      (3) Cystic – gallbladder

3. Splenic – spleen, pancreas
   d. Left gastroepiploic – greater curve of stomach from left to right

I. Superior mesenteric (color orange)

Arises from the aorta a short distance inferior to the celiac trunk; supplies part of the duodenum, all of the small intestine, cecum, appendix, ascending colon, and the proximal half of the transverse colon.
4. Inferior pancreaticoduodenal
5. Jejunal branches
6. Ileal branches
7. Ileocolic
   a. Appendicular – appendix
8. Right colic – ascending colon
9. Middle colic – transverse colon

J. Inferior mesenteric (color red-orange)

Arises from the aorta posterior, or just distal, to the duodenum; supplies the distal half of the transverse colon and the descending and sigmoid colon.
10. Left colic – distal half of the transverse colon; descending colon
11. Sigmoid – sigmoid colon
12. Superior rectal (hemorrhoidal) – continuation of the inferior mesenteric into the pelvis; supplies the superior portion of the rectum

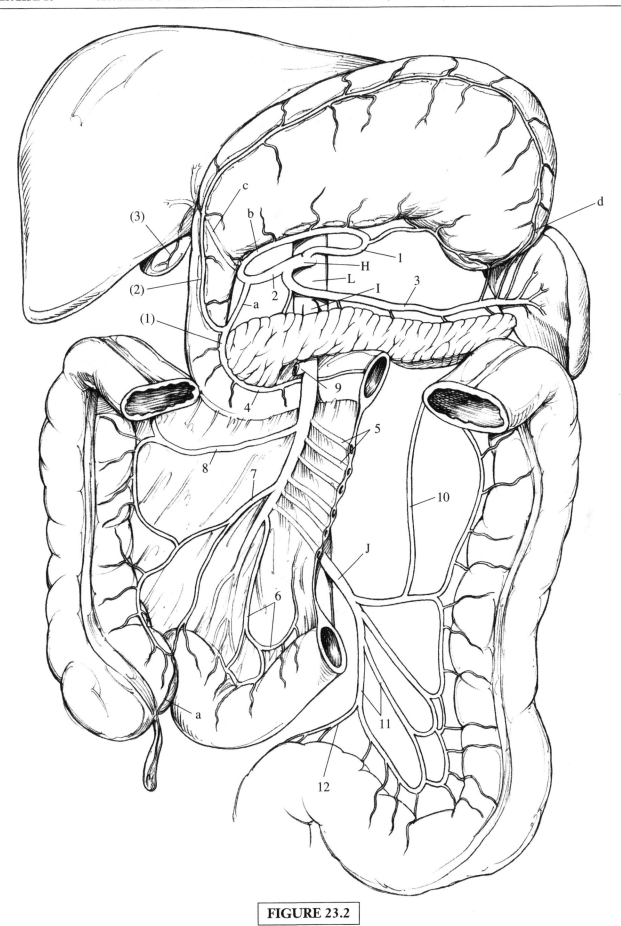

FIGURE 23.2

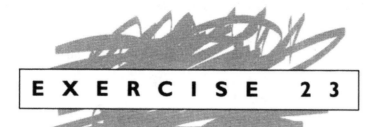

Arterial Supply and Venous Drainage of the Thorax, Abdomen, and Pelvis

Letters A–C represent paired branches to glands (FIGURE 23.3).

A. Suprarenal – adrenal glands
B. Renal – kidneys
C. Gonadal – generally arise superior to the origin of the inferior mesenteric ovarian (female); testicular (male)

Letters D–F represent branches to body wall structures.

D. Inferior phrenic – inferior surface of the diaphragm
E. Lumbar – usually four pairs, to muscles and skin of the back; psoas major and quadratus lumborum
F. Median sacral – a direct continuation of the aorta; courses on the ventral surface of the sacrum

BIFURCATION OF THE AORTA

The aorta bifurcates into the *common iliac arteries* (G) (color sky blue) at the level of the fourth lumbar vertebra (FIGURE 23.4). These then split into *internal* (H) (color blue) and *external iliac arteries* (I) (color violet) at the level of the fifth lumbar or first sacral vertebra. The internal iliac arteries pass into the pelvis to supply muscles and viscera while the external iliacs continue into the lower limb.

Internal Iliac

J. Iliolumbar – psoas major, quadratus lumborum, ilium
K. Lateral sacral
L. Obturator – pelvic muscles, hip joint, anterior and medial thigh

1. Pubic
2. Acetabular
3. Anterior
4. Posterior
M. Superior gluteal – muscles of the gluteal region
N. Inferior gluteal – muscles of the gluteal region
O. Umbilical – a continuation of the internal iliac; a remnant, only partially patent
Visceral branches
5. Uterine
   a. Vaginal
   b. Tubal
6. Middle rectal
7. Internal pudendal
   c. Inferior rectal
   d. Perineal
   e. Urethral
   f. Penile/clitoral

External Iliac

P. Inferior epigastric – abdominal wall, peritoneum, cremaster muscle
8. Cremasteric (artery of the round ligament of the uterus)
Q. Deep iliac circumflex – psoas major, iliacus, sartorius, tensor fascia latae

After giving off the deep iliac circumflex artery, the external iliac passes deep to the inguinal ligament and continues in the thigh as the femoral artery.

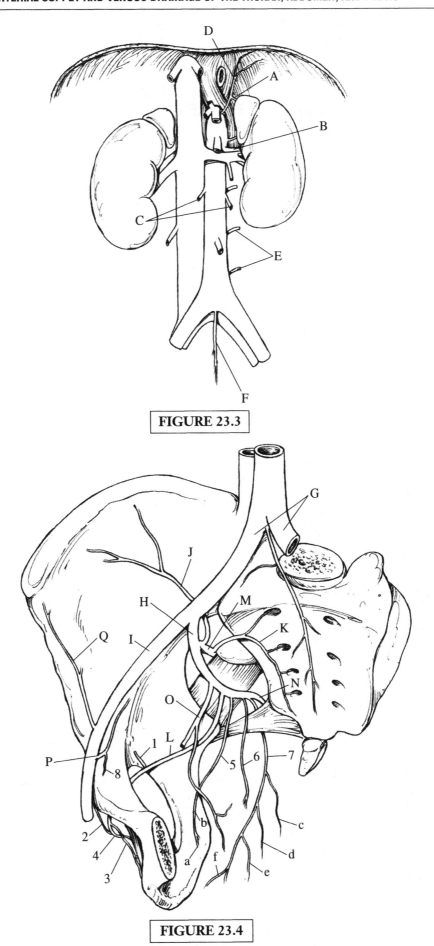

FIGURE 23.3

FIGURE 23.4

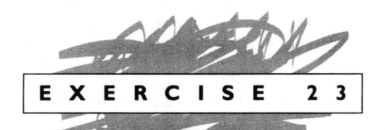

Arterial Supply and Venous Drainage of the Thorax, Abdomen, and Pelvis

VISCERAL VEINS OF THE PELVIS AND ABDOMEN

Venous drainage of the gastrointestinal viscera does not pass directly to the inferior vena cava, but instead passes through the *hepatic portal system* (FIGURE 23.5). (Color the four veins listed below brown.)

A. Inferior mesenteric
B. Splenic
C. Superior mesenteric
D. Portal vein

The portal vein accepts this venous blood and passes it to the liver. In the liver the veins break up into a network of *sinusoidal capillaries* (E) and exit via *hepatic veins* (F). These veins empty into the *inferior vena cava* (G).

SYSTEMIC VEINS OF THE PELVIS AND ABDOMEN

These veins (FIGURE 23.6) usually accompany the arteries and are given the same names. They drain into the inferior vena cava which is formed at the level of the fourth lumbar vertebra by the union of the two *common iliac veins* (H), each of which, in turn, has received drainage from the *internal* (I) and *external iliac veins* (J). Other veins draining into the inferior vena cava.

K. Lumbar – usually four pairs
L. Gonadal – right side only; the left empties into the renal vein
M. Renal
N. Suprarenal – right side only; the left empties into the renal vein
O. Inferior phrenic

SYSTEMIC VEINS OF THE THORAX

Azygos Venous System

The azygos system of veins (FIGURE 23.7) drains most of the thorax. The *azygos* (L., alone) *vein* (P) ascends the anterolateral surface of the vertebral column after its formation by a union of the right subcostal vein and an ascending lumbar vein. An asymmetrical 'partner', the *hemiazygos vein* (Q), arises and ascends similarly. This vein is usually considerably smaller. In their ascent both receive blood from the *posterior intercostal veins* (R). The hemiazygos may also receive drainage from an *accessory hemiazygos vein* (S). The hemiazygos ends by crossing the anterior surface of the vertebral column to join the azygos, which then empties into the superior vena cava just before its entrance into the right atrium.

Other Venous Drainage

The paired internal thoracic veins empty into the brachiocephalic veins. These drain the areas supplied by the branches of the internal thoracic artery. The veins are named accordingly: superior epigastric, musculophrenic, and anterior intercostal.

❓ FOR REVIEW AND THOUGHT

Why the need for the hepatic portal system?

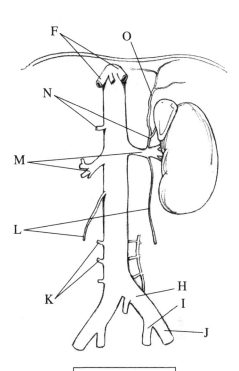

FIGURE 23.6

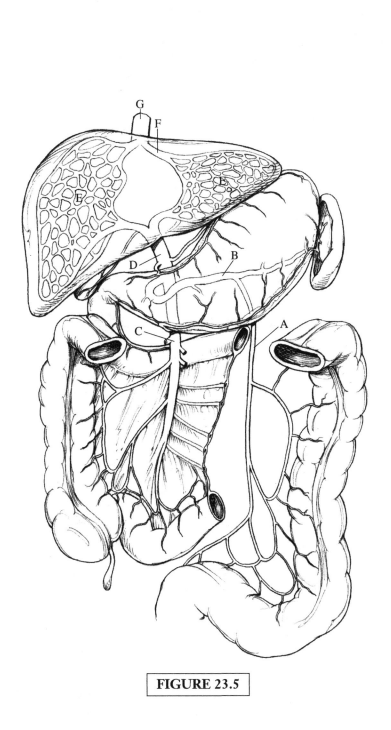

FIGURE 23.5

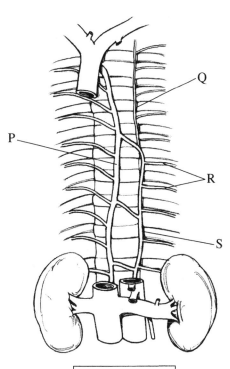

FIGURE 23.7

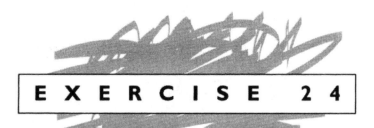

Arterial Supply and Venous Drainage of the Lower Limb

After passing deep to the inguinal ligament the external iliac artery becomes the *femoral artery* (A) (FIGURE 24.1). It will continue as such until reaching the adductor hiatus.

FEMORAL ARTERY (A)

A_1. Superficial and deep external pudendal
A_2. Superficial iliac circumflex
B. Deep femoral (Profunda femoris) – in the femoral triangle (color yellow)
   1. Medial femoral circumflex – head and neck of the femur and the superior 1/3 of the thigh (color yellow-green)
     a. Deep
     b. Ascending
     c. Transverse
     d. Acetabular
   2. Lateral femoral circumflex – same area of distribution as the medial
     e. Ascending
     f. Descending
     g. Transverse
   3. Perforating arteries – posterior thigh

Upon reaching the adductor hiatus the femoral artery becomes the *popliteal artery* (C) (FIGURE 24.2).

POPLITEAL ARTERY

D. Muscular branches – adductor magnus; hamstrings
E. Descending genicular
F. Superior genicular – knee joint proximal to femoral condyles
   4. Lateral
   5. Medial
G. Inferior genicular – knee joint distal to femoral condyles
   6. Lateral
   7. Medial

Upon reaching the inferior border of the popliteus muscle the popliteal artery splits into the *anterior* (H) and *posterior* (I) *tibial arteries*.

ANTERIOR TIBIAL ARTERY

The anterior tibial artery courses on the anterior surface of the interosseous membrane.

J. Anterior tibial recurrent
K. Anterior malleolar
   8. Lateral
   9. Medial
L. Dorsalis pedis – the continuation of the anterior tibial into the foot
   10. Arcuate artery – arches across the bases of the metatarsals from medial to lateral
   11. Dorsal metatarsal arteries
     h. dorsal digital arteries
     i. deep plantar branch – for communication with the plantar arch

POSTERIOR TIBIAL ARTERY

The posterior tibial is found on the posteromedial side of the leg.

M. Peroneal – deep calf muscles, peroneal muscles

After passing posterior to the medial malleolus it splits into two branches to the plantar surface of the foot.

N. Medial plantar – medial side of foot and first digit
O. Lateral plantar – passes obliquely across the sole to reach the base of the fifth metatarsal, then arches medially and anastomoses with the deep branch of the dorsalis pedis to form the *plantar arch* (P). This arch then gives off plantar metatarsal and digital branches

❓ FOR REVIEW AND THOUGHT

The branches of the medial and lateral femoral circumflex arteries are of great significance to the integrity of the coxofemoral joint. These vessels supply the neck and head of the femur. Decreased blood flow through these vessels due to age, disease, etc. may compromise the strength of the femoral neck resulting in fracture. This is an all too common occurrence in the elderly!

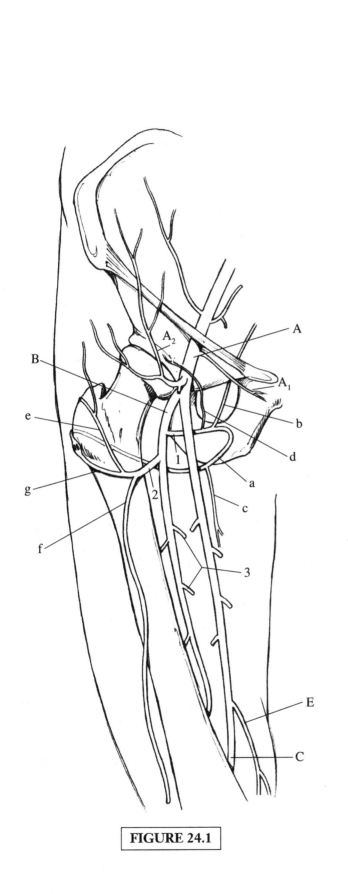

FIGURE 24.1

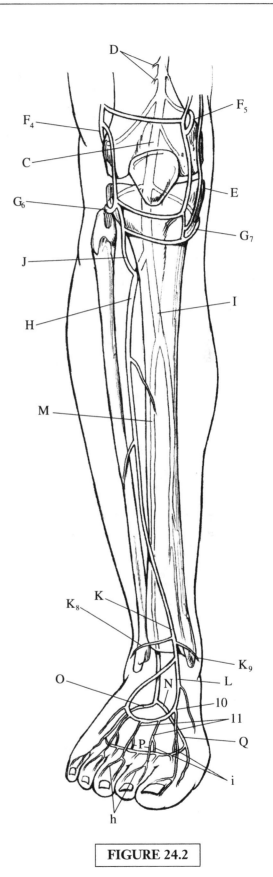

FIGURE 24.2

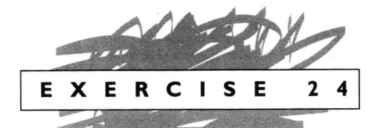

EXERCISE 24

Arterial Supply and Venous Drainage of the Lower Limb

VENOUS DRAINAGE OF THE LOWER LIMB

The venous drainage of the lower limb is organized much like that of the upper limb. Deep veins accompany the arteries (venae comitantes) and have the same names. A system of superficial veins is also present (FIGURES 24.3a and 24.3b).

Great Saphenous Vein

The *great saphenous vein* (A) originates on the medial side of the dorsal venous arch of the foot. It ascends immediately anterior to the medial malleolus, along the medial side of the leg, and passes posterior to the medial tibial and femoral condyles. It continues along the medial side of the thigh to drain into the femoral vein in the femoral triangle (color blue).

Lesser Saphenous Vein

The *lesser saphenous vein* (B) (color brown) begins on the lateral side of the dorsal venous arch of the foot, passes posterior to the lateral malleolus, and ascends along the posterior leg to empty into the popliteal vein.

PERFORATING VEINS (C)

These connect the superficial and deep venous systems and have valves to allow flow from superficial to deep. Venous return to the thorax (against the force of gravity) is aided by muscular contraction 'milking' blood against this force. If these valves should become incompetent venous flow is not as efficient from superficial to deep, resulting in a reverse flow and pooling of blood in superficial veins. Such pooling is often shown by tortuous tributaries of the great saphenous vein: **varicose veins.** Varicose veins are common in older persons and in those engaged in sedentary occupations.

❓ FOR REVIEW AND THOUGHT

Venous cutdowns of the great saphenous vein are used to "bypass" occlusions of the coronary arteries!

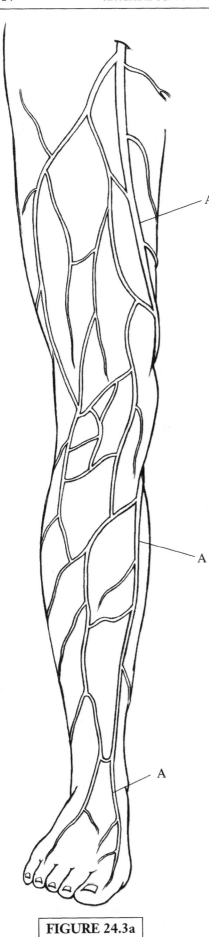

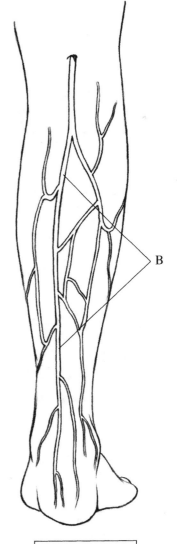

FIGURE 24.3a

FIGURE 24.3b

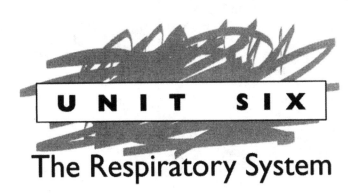

UNIT SIX

The Respiratory System

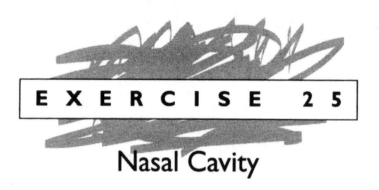

Nasal Cavity

In this section we will describe structures and organs involved in speech and respiration. Quiet respiration usually occurs via the nose. The mouth becomes involved in respiration associated with more intensive levels of activity such as aerobic exercise or conditions of disease or illness.

The nasal cavity is divided by a septum of both bone and cartilage (FIGURES 25.1 and 25.2). The bony portion is formed by the *perpendicular plate of the ethmoid* (A) and the *vomer* (B). The *cartilaginous portion* (C) fills the gap anterior to these two bony processes. The lateral walls of each nostril include the mucous membrane covered *superior* (D), *middle* (E), and *inferior conchae* (F); and an associated *meatus* (D_1, E_1, and F_1) inferior to each. A small portion of this mucosa on the superior concha, just inferior to the cribriform plate of the ethmoid bone, is described as the *olfactory region* (color yellow). The remainder of the mucosa is designated as the *respiratory region* (color orange).

Mucous membrane-lined paranasal sinuses are intimately associated with the nasal cavity (FIGURE 25.3). The *ethmoidal* (G), *frontal* (H), and *maxillary* (I), and *sphenoidal* (J) sinuses certainly impact breathing and speech, to which anyone who has had a cold, or suffers from allergies, can attest. Mucous secreted in these sinuses passes into the nasal cavity via meatuses (openings) on the lateral walls of the cavity.

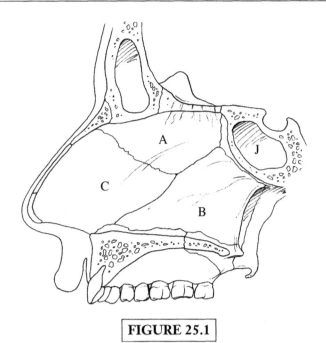

FIGURE 25.1

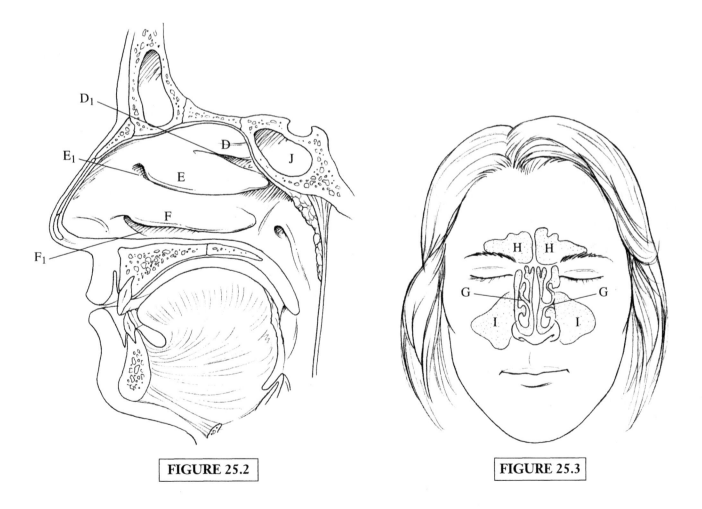

FIGURE 25.2   **FIGURE 25.3**

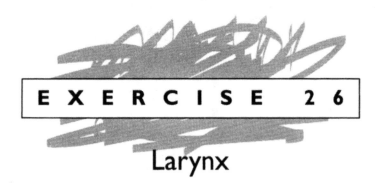

Larynx

The *larynx* (A) (FIGURE 26.1) is found posterior and inferior to the nasal cavity in the anterior portion of the pharynx. The larynx consists of several cartilages guarding the inlet of the respiratory tree and involved in the process of producing sound. The *thyroid cartilage* (B) *(FIGURE 26.2a-c)* shows paired *laminae* (C_1) on each anterolateral surface, meeting in a midline *prominence* (C_2): **the Adam's apple**. The midline also shows a large *superior thyroid notch* (C_3). Other portions of the thyroid cartilage include the *oblique line* (C_4), and *superior* (C_5) and *inferior* (C_6) *horns*. The thyroid cartilage is connected with the hyoid bone superiorly via the *thyrohyoid membrane* (D) and inferiorly with the cricoid cartilage via the *cricothyroid ligament* (E). The *epiglottic cartilage* (F) takes attachment from the internal surface of the thyroid cartilage. This serves in protecting the entrance to the larynx during swallowing.

The inferior horns of the thyroid cartilage articulate with the lateral surfaces of the *cricoid cartilage* (G). This articulation allows both flexion/extension as well as anterior/posterior gliding. The cricoid cartilage is shaped like a signet ring, with the wide portion, the *lamina* (G_1), posterior. The cricoid cartilage also articulates with a pair of *arytenoid cartilages* (H); each with an *articular surface* (H_1). The arytenoid cartilages are pyramidal in shape and each has an *apex* (H_2), a *base* (H_3), and *vocal* (H_4) and *muscular processes* (H_5).

The relationship of the arytenoid cartilages to the cricoid cartilage is central to the process of vocation. *Vocal folds (chords)* (I) (color red-orange) pass from the vocal processes of the arytenoid cartilages to the deep surface of the thyroid cartilage. These are the free edges of the laryngeal mucous membrane. The opening between these folds, leading to the trachea, is the *glottis* (J). Just superior to the vocal folds another pair of mucosal lined folds is present, the *vestibular folds* (K), sometimes called the false vocal chords.

A number of muscles function in the positioning of the cartilages, and therefore the vocal folds; or in tensing the folds.

cricothyroid (L) – from the external surface of the cricoid cartilage to the internal and external surfaces of the thyroid lamina; function to tense the vocal folds (color red).

posterior cricoarytenoid (M) – from the laminae of the cricoid cartilage to the muscular processes of the arytenoid cartilages; function in abducting the vocal folds (opening the glottis) (color green).

lateral cricoarytenoid (N) – from the lateral surface of the cricoid cartilage to the muscular processes of the arytenoid cartilages; function in adducting the vocal folds (closing the glottis) (color blue).

transverse arytenoid (O) – from the posterior surface of one arytenoid to the same surface of the other; function in adducting these cartilages and closing the glottis (color violet).

vocalis (P) – from the inner surface of the thyroid cartilage to the vocal process of the arytenoid cartilage; aids in providing varying amounts of tension on the folds to alter the quality of vibration (color sky blue).

Inferior to the vocal folds is the *laryngeal cavity* (Q) and the beginning of the trachea (color brown).

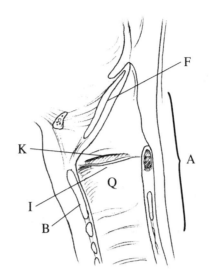

FIGURE 26.1

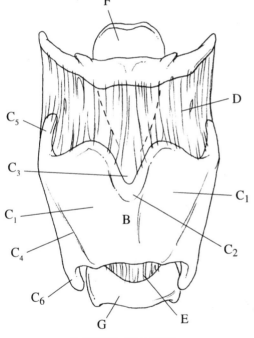

FIGURE 26.2a

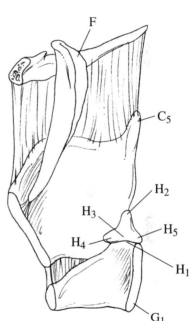

FIGURE 26.2b

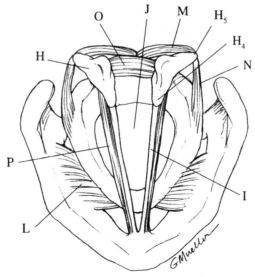

FIGURE 26.2c

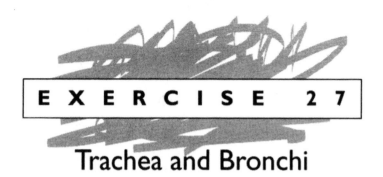

EXERCISE 27

Trachea and Bronchi

TRACHEA

The *trachea* (A) (FIGURE 27.1a and 27.1b) descends inferiorly from the larynx for about 12 cm. The lumen of the trachea is maintained by incomplete c-shaped *cartilaginous rings* (B) on the anterior and lateral aspects of the tracheal wall. The esophagus lies immediately posterior to the trachea, accounting for the absence of these cartilaginous structures on this surface. The posterior wall of the trachea is a flattened membrane that can stretch during the passage of food in the esophagus. The length of its course is approximately 12 cm.

A structure in intimate relationship with the trachea is the *thyroid gland* (C). The paired lobes of this gland lie on either side of the first four tracheal cartilages and meet in the midline via the *isthmus* (D) at about the third cartilage. Surgical incision through the midline of the anterior neck (tracheotomy) for purposes of reestablishing an airway in the case of laryngeal obstruction is performed just inferior to the isthmus.

The trachea ends at approximately the level of T_4 by bifurcating into the *left* (E) and *right* (F) *primary bronchi*. At this bifurcation a sharp crest presents itself in the tracheal lumen, the *carina (keel)* (G), coursing anteroposteriorly between the orifices of the bronchi. This structure is of significance because its mucous membrane is quite sensitive and is intimately involved in the cough reflex.

BRONCHI

The bifurcation is not perfectly symmetrical. The right bronchus continues on a straighter course than that of the left and is, therefore, the more common site of lodged matter. Each primary bronchus splits into lobar bronchi in a predictable pattern based upon the lobe of the lung to which they pass (FIGURE 27.1a).

The first branch off the right primary bronchus is the *right superior lobar bronchus* (H), which in turn yields the following bronchi:

apical (H_1) (color yellow),
posterior (H_2) (orange), and
anterior (H_3) (red-orange).

The next branch off the right primary bronchus is the *right middle lobar* (I) with two branches:

lateral (I_1) (red) and
medial (I_2) (yellow-green).

The right primary bronchus terminates as the *right inferior lobar bronchus* (J) with five branches:

superior segmental (J_1) (green),
medial basal (J_2) (sky blue),
anterior basal (J_3) (blue),
lateral basal (J_4) (brown), and
posterior basal (J_5) (light brown).

The left primary bronchus splits into superior and inferior lobar bronchi; again with a predictable pattern of branches destined to specific lung segments. The *left superior lobar bronchus* (K) yields:

apicoposterior (K_1) (color yellow),
anterior (K_2) (orange),
superior lingular (K_3) (red-orange), and
inferior lingular (K_4) (red).

The *left inferior lobar bronchus* (L) is the origin of five bronchi supplying the inferior portion of the lung. These branches are:

superior (L_1) (yellow-green),
medial basal (L_2) (green),
anterior basal (L3) (sky blue),
lateral basal (L_4) (blue), and
posterior basal (L_5) (violet).

❓ FOR REVIEW AND THOUGHT

Reinforce the distribution of the bronchi by outlining the boundaries of their pulmonary segments (lobes) (FIGURE 27.1c and 27.1d) in the same color.

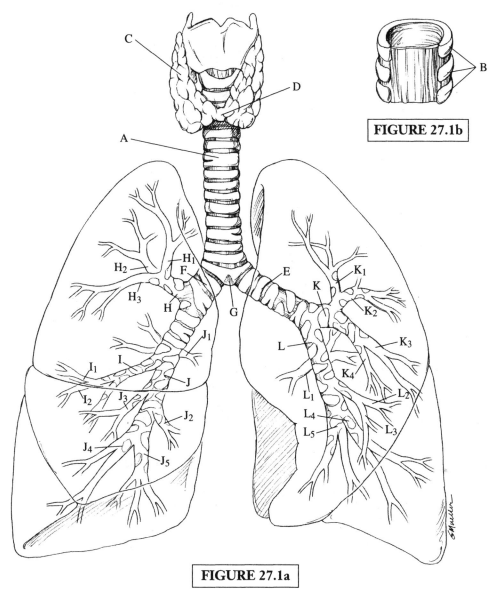

FIGURE 27.1b

FIGURE 27.1a

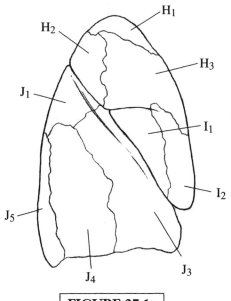

FIGURE 27.1c

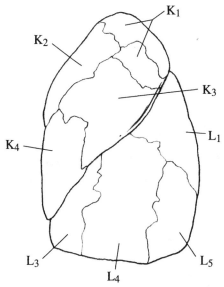

FIGURE 27.1d

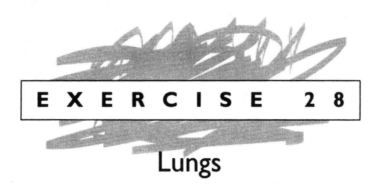

EXERCISE 28

Lungs

A view of the complete lung shows the lobes clearly (FIGURE 28.1a). The superior most tip of the lung is the *apex* (A) and the most inferior portion the *base* (B). Each lung is covered intimately with *visceral pleura* (C) (color brown) which passes into the depths of the fissures between lobes. Each lung also shows *lateral* (D), *medial* (E), and *diaphragmatic* (F) *surfaces*. The walls of the pleural cavity and the superior surface of the *thoracic diaphragm* (G) are lined with *parietal pleura* (H) (color black) (FIGURE 28.1b).

Note the fissures delineating the lobes of each lung. The right lung presents *oblique* (I) and *horizontal fissures* (J) and therefore shows three lobes; while the left shows only an *oblique fissure* (K) and has two lobes. These fissures are seen on the medial surface as well (FIGURE 28.1c and 28.1d). On the medial surface find the *root of the lung* (L); the point of entry/exit of primary bronchi and vessels. The left lung shows two characteristics associated with the position of the heart: the *cardiac notch* (M) and the *cardiac impression* (N).

FIGURE 28.1e presents a cross sectional view of the heart and lungs in situ. The entire thoracic cavity and its structures are lined with pleura. *Parietal pleura* (O) covers the wall of the thorax and is continuous at the root of the lung with *visceral pleura* (P). The visceral pleura continues into the depths of the fissures between lobes as well. Note that visceral pleura is also reflected upon the external surface of the pericardium. Color the pleuras as described above (visceral brown, parietal black).

The *pleural cavity* (Q) is a potential space between the visceral and parietal pleuras. In breathing the moist pleural layers are adherent and move together. Inspiration causes an expansion of intrathoracic volume and a resultant decrease in intrathoracic pressure, leading to flow of air into the lungs. Expiration is the converse of this.

❓ FOR REVIEW AND THOUGHT

What is the nerve supply to the thoracoabdominal diaphragm?

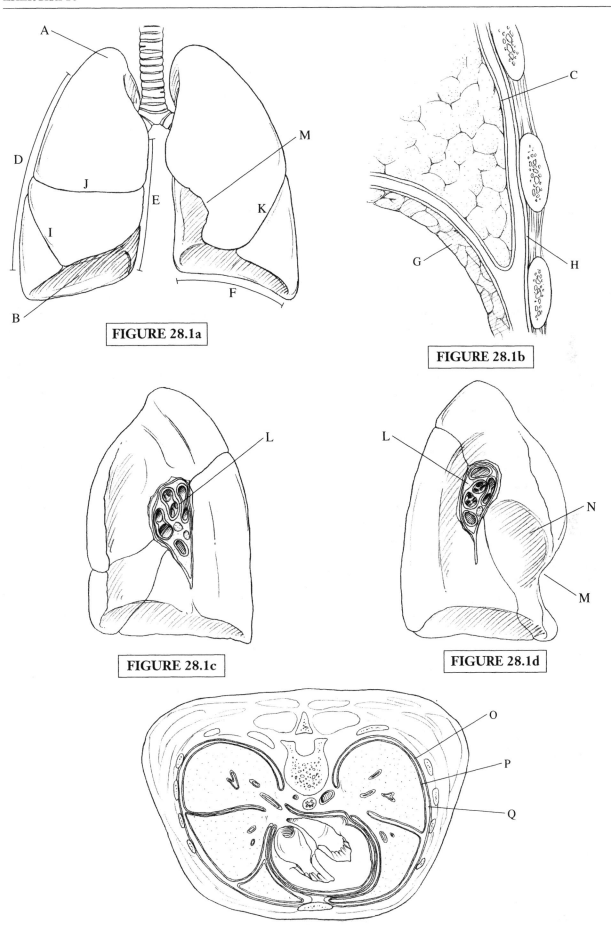

FIGURE 28.1a

FIGURE 28.1b

FIGURE 28.1c

FIGURE 28.1d

FIGURE 28.1e

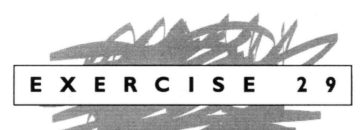

EXERCISE 29

Thoracoabdominal Diaphragm

The musculotendinous *thoracoabdominal diaphragm* (A) (FIGURE 29.1) partitions the thoracic and abdominal cavities and is concave inferiorly (abdominal surface). The muscular portion of the diaphragm shows three distinct contributors: *sternal* (A_1) (color orange), *costal* (A_2) (color red-orange), and *vertebral* (A_3) (color red). The sternal portion is quite small with muscle fibers passing from the deep surface of the xiphoid process. The costal portion is much larger with muscle fibers passing radially from the internal surface of the inferior six pair of ribs. The vertebral portion passes from the lumbar vertebrae via two *crura* ($B_{1,2}$) and the *arcuate ligaments*: paired *lateral* (C), paired *medial* (D), and a solitary *median* (E) (color these ligaments green, sky blue, and violet, respectively)

The *right* (B_1) and *left* (B_2) crura ascend from the anterior longitudinal ligament of the superior three lumbar vertebrae. The *median arcuate ligament* (E) is formed by the union of the medial portions of each crus. The aorta passes deep to this ligament, and between the crura, on its way into the abdomen. The fibers of the right crus continue to ascend to surround the *esophageal hiatus* (F). The medial arcuate ligaments arch between the crura and the transverse process of the first lumbar vertebra. The psoas major muscle lies deep to this arch. The lateral arcuate ligaments overlie the superior portion of the quadratus lumborum muscle; passing from the tip of the first or second lumbar vertebra to the 12th rib.

The portion of the diaphragm attaching to the lateral arcuate ligament is often thin, due to a lack of muscle fibers. This area, the *vertebrocostal triangle* (G), is a site for potential herniation of abdominal contents into the thorax; especially so on the left side.

The aponeurotic central portion of the diaphragm is the *central tendon* (H) (color yellow) into which the muscle fibers of the diaphragm attach. The *foramen for passage of the inferior vena cava* (I) is found in the central tendon.

❓ FOR REVIEW AND THOUGHT

How many structures pass through the thoracoabdominal diaphragm? Be careful about quickly saying three: the aorta passes posterior to the diaphragm!

In heavy exercise what effect might diaphragmatic contraction have on venous return to the heart?

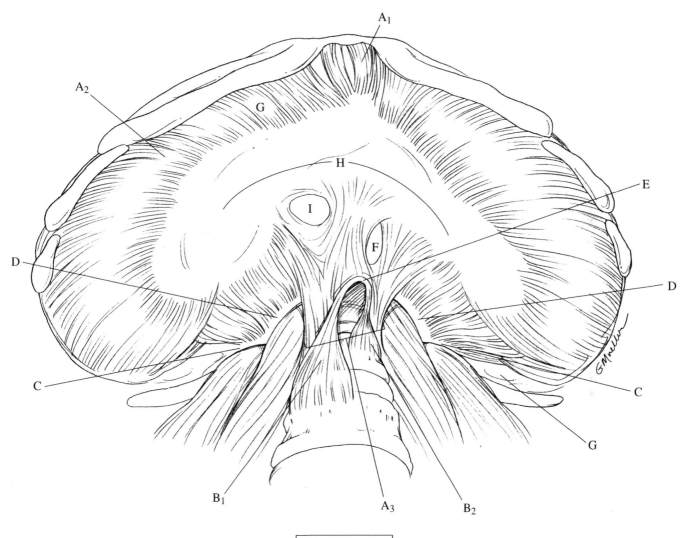

FIGURE 29.1

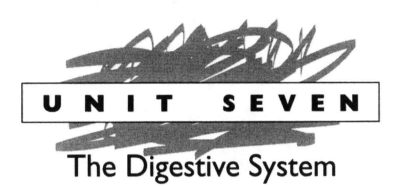

UNIT SEVEN

The Digestive System

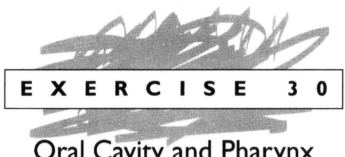

Oral Cavity and Pharynx

MOUTH

The process of digestion begins the moment food enters the *oral cavity* (A) (FIGURE 30.1a and 30.1b), defined as the space bounded anteriorly by the lips, laterally by the cheeks, and posteriorly by the entrance into the oropharynx. To be precise the oral cavity proper is bounded by the teeth. The area between the teeth and cheeks is the vestibule, or *buccal cavity* (B). The roof of the oral cavity is formed anteriorly by the *hard palate* (C) and posteriorly by the *soft palate* (D) and its midline projection, the *uvula* (E). The entrance into the oropharynx is via an opening called the faucial isthmus, found between the *palatoglossal arches* (F). Slightly posterior are the *palatopharyngeal arches* (G). (These arches are formed by underlying palatoglossal and palatopharyngeal muscles and their covering epithelium.) Both function to lower the soft palate.

Tucked neatly between these two arches are the *palatine tonsils* (H) (color yellow). A third "arch-like" landmark is the *pterygomandibular raphe* (I), a tendinous structure passing from the pterygoid hamulus of the medial pterygoid plate to the mylohyoid line of the mandible. This raphe serves as the site of attachment for the buccinator and superior pharyngeal constrictor muscles.

Three pairs of *salivary glands* (FIGURE 30.1c) are intimately involved in initiating digestion. The *sublingual glands* (J) (color orange) are found on the floor of the mouth between the mandible and the genioglossus muscle. They open into the floor of the mouth via numerous small ducts. The *submandibular glands* (K) (color red-orange) lie adjacent and deep to the mylohyoid muscle. Each empties into the anterior portion of the floor of the mouth via a duct beneath the frenulum of the tongue. The *parotid glands* (L) (color red) are tucked posterior to the ramus of the mandible. Each opens into the oral cavity via a duct that runs on the external surface of the masseter muscle, pierces the buccinator muscle, and opens on the inside of the cheek near the second molar. The mylohyoid muscle (M) elevates the floor of the mouth and tongue.

TONGUE

The tongue aids in the initiation of digestion (with the aid of the buccinator muscle and the muscles of mastication, first by positioning food between the teeth and finally by pushing a bolus of food to the back of the oral cavity for swallowing. Some important extrinsic muscles are the *genioglossus* (N) (color yellow-green), *hyoglossus* (O) (color green), and *styloglossus* (P) (color sky blue); shown in FIGURE 30.1d. What are the proximal attachments of these three muscles? A variety of intrinsic longitudinal and transverse muscles function in changing the shape of the tongue. These aid somewhat in digestion but are most intimately involved in the ability to make sounds and develop speech.

❓ FOR REVIEW AND THOUGHT

Return to page 86 and the discussion of the hyoid bone and associated muscles. How might these be involved in the initiation of digestion?

Have you ever attempted to learn a foreign language? What makes the vowels and ch's auf Deutsch, or the rolling r's de Espanol so difficult to learn? Would it be easier if learned earlier in life?

PHARYNX

The pharynx is that part of the throat located posterior to the oral and nasal cavities. It extends from the *fornix* (Q) superiorly to the beginning of the esophagus. It is described as having nasal, oral, and laryngeal portions (FIGURES 30.1a, 30.1b, 30.1c, and 30.1d). The *palatine tonsil* (adenoid) (R) is found on the posterior wall of the fornix, in the nasal portion. The *auditory (Eustachian) tube* (S) also opens into the nasal portion. The laryngeal portion features the *epiglottis* (T), a lid-like cartilaginous structure guarding the entrance to the larynx during swallowing.

The posterolateral muscular wall of the pharynx (FIGURE 30.1d) is composed mainly of three paired constrictors all having distal attachment on a posterior midline connective tissue seam: the *pharyngeal raphe* (U) (color black). The *superior constrictor* (V) (color blue) includes four portions with their proximal attachments on the medial pterygoid plate and hamulus (pterygopharyngeal), the pterygomandibular raphe (buccopharyngeal), the mylohyoid line of the mandible (mylopharyngeal), and the intrinsic muscles of the tongue (glossopharyngeal). The *middle constrictor* (W) (color violet) is comprised of two portions; one from the lesser horn of the hyoid bone (chondropharyngeal) and one from the greater horn (ceratopharyngeal). The *inferior constrictor* (X) (color brown) also has two portions; (thyropharyngeal) from the oblique line of the thyroid cartilage and (cricopharyngeal) from the cricoid cartilage.

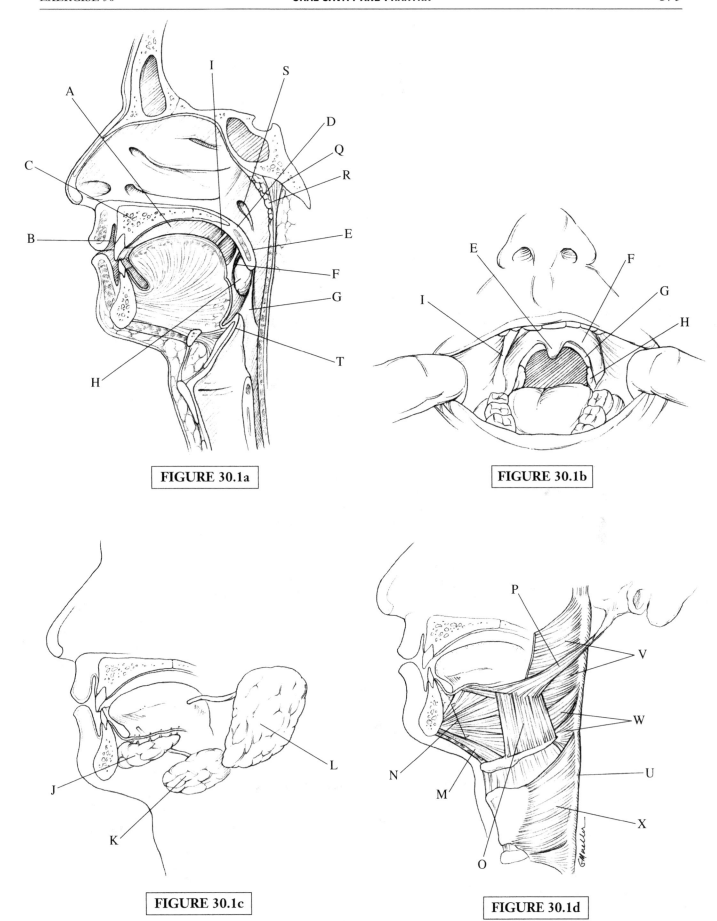

FIGURE 30.1a

FIGURE 30.1b

FIGURE 30.1c

FIGURE 30.1d

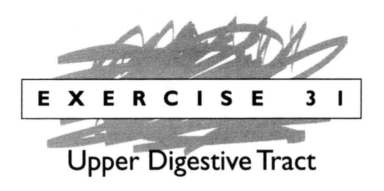

Upper Digestive Tract

ESOPHAGUS

The esophagus (FIGURE 31.1a) begins the alimentary canal and runs a course of approximately 25 cm beginning at the level of the cricoid cartilage (C_6), passing through the diaphragm, and terminating at its entrance into the stomach. It is described as having cervical, thoracic, and abdominal portions.

We are about to venture into the abdominal cavity and discussion about a variety of important and complex organs. Before beginning this journey we need to address the concepts of the linings of the abdomen.

FIGURE 31.1b presents a schematic view of the manner in which various organs are situated within the abdomen. The abdominal cavity shows both *parietal* (A) (on the body wall) and *visceral* (on the organ) *peritoneum* (B). Parietal peritoneum (color orange) lines the body wall and dorsally is reflected onto the viscera of the gastrointestinal tract as a double layer. Such a double layer of visceral peritoneum is a *mesentery* (C) (color red-orange) and is common and complex in the abdomen. It is through such mesenteries that nerves and vascular supply reach the organ. Visceral peritoneum (color red) is intimately attached to the external surface of a number of abdominal organs. Organs without a mesentery, such as the kidneys (represented in FIGURE 31.1b), are described as being retroperitoneal. In all cases this does not literally mean 'behind the peritoneum', but does mean 'without a mesentery'. As you study the organs of the abdomen and pelvis determine whether they are with or without a mesentery and maintain the coloring scheme we have just presented.

STOMACH

The entrance of the esophagus into the stomach (FIGURE 31.1c) occurs at the *cardiac orifice* (D), approximately 1/3 distance from the superior end of the organ. The portion of the stomach superior to the entrance of the esophagus is the *fundus* (E). The central portion is the *body* (F) and the most distal is the *pyloric* (G) portion. At this end the stomach is continuous with the duodenum via the *pyloric orifice* (H) controlled by a circular layer of smooth muscle, the *pyloric sphincter* (I) (color yellow-green).

The stomach is also described by its curves. The *greater curvature* (J) (trace in green) is along the left and inferior borders and the *lesser curvature* (K) (trace in sky blue) along the right and superior borders.

The stomach features two mesenteries attaching along these borders. The *lesser omentum* (L) connects the liver with the proximal duodenum and the lesser curve of the stomach. The *greater omentum* (M) hangs like an apron from the greater curvature, obscuring the small intestine. Inferiorly it is attached to the anterior surface of the transverse colon.

DUODENUM

This "C-shaped" structure (FIGURE 31.1d) at the origin of the small intestine has four parts: *superior* (N) (color violet), *descending* (O) (color light brown), *horizontal* (P) (color brown), *and ascending* (Q) (color black). Several important structures open into the descending portion. The *major duodenal papilla* (the Ampulla of Vater) (R) presents the joint opening of the *greater pancreatic* (S) and *common bile ducts* (T). Just superior to this a *minor duodenal papilla* (U) for the opening of the *accessory pancreatic duct* (V) is sometimes found.

The duodenum ends at the *duodenojejunal flexure* (W) where the ascending portion meets the jejunum. At this point a *suspensory muscle of the duodenum* (X) anchors this junction to the right crus of the thoracic diaphragm. Interestingly, this structure, not truly a muscle, is composed of skeletal muscle, elastic fibers, and smooth muscle.

❓ FOR REVIEW AND THOUGHT

Take a few moments and review the concepts of the various types of peritoneum. Become comfortable with terms like retroperitoneal, mesentery, and omentum.

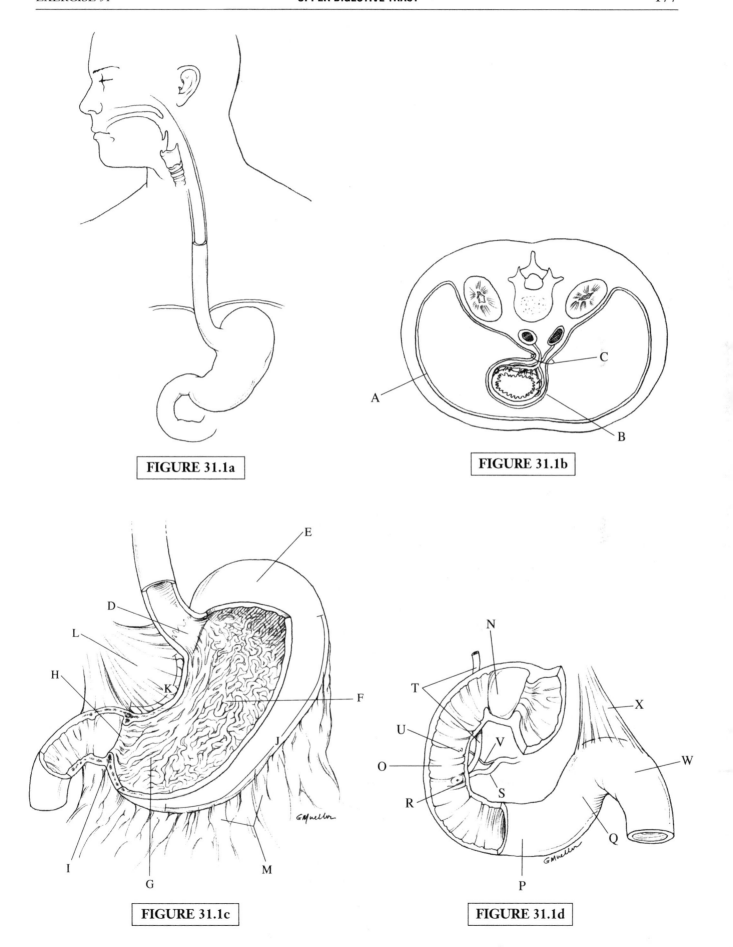

FIGURE 31.1a

FIGURE 31.1b

FIGURE 31.1c

FIGURE 31.1d

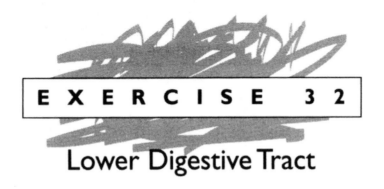

EXERCISE 32

Lower Digestive Tract

JEJUNUM AND ILEUM

The *jejunum* (A) (FIGURE 32.1a) begins at the duodeno-jejunal flexure and comprises approximately 40% of the remaining length of the small intestine. No clear junction is shown between the jejunum and the terminal portion of the small intestine, the *ileum* (B); the remaining 60%. The ileum joins the beginning of the large intestine at the *ileocecal orifice* (C).

LARGE INTESTINE

The large intestine (colon) surrounds the small intestine on three sides like an inverted U and presents several identifying features. Three longitudinal bands of muscle, *the teniae coli* (D), arranged 120° apart, course the length of the organ (color these yellow). These are absent on the jejunum and ileum and therefore serve to clearly identify the colon. *Haustra* (E), appear segmentally and are aligned with attachments of the teniae coli to the exterior surface of the colon. *Appendices epiploicae* (F), small pouches of fat-filled peritoneum, are seen throughout the colon but are most prominent in the sigmoid portion.

The ileocecal orifice (FIGURE 32.1b) is situated at the superior end of the *cecum* (G) (color orange), a blind pouch at the inferior end of the *ascending colon* (H). Two thickened lips of the ileal wall project slightly into the cecum as the *ileocecal valve* (I). The cecum is, of itself, insignificant, but it does include an appendage, the *vermiform appendix* (J) (color red), attaching inferior to the ileocecal junction. The appendix is usually about 9 cm long and contains abundant lymphatic tissue. The anterior teniae coli leads directly to the appendix. Interestingly the appendix has its own mesentery, the *mesoappendix* (K).

The ascending colon passes retroperitoneally to a point just inferior to the liver where it bends sharply to the left to become the *transverse colon* (L) (FIGURE 32.1a). This bend is the *hepatic flexure* (M), also called the right colic flexure. The transverse colon is embedded within the greater omentum and also has its own mesentery: the *transverse mesocolon* (N). The transverse colon passes to the left toward the spleen where it again bends sharply to become the *descending colon* (O). This is the *splenic flexure* (P), also called the left colic flexure. The descending colon, like its ascending counterpart is retroperitoneal. It continues as the *sigmoid colon* (Q), a portion variable in length and named by its resemblance to the Greek letter sigma. It connects the colon to the rectum and has a mesentery, the sigmoid mesocolon.

RECTUM

The *rectum* (R) (FIGURES 32.1c and 32.1d) is usually about 15 cm long and has neither teniae coli or a mesentery. In its course it presents two flexures. The first is an anteriorly concave *sacral flexure* (S) to conform with the curve of the sacrum; the second an anteriorly convex *perineal flexure* (T) for passage through the pelvic diaphragm and continuation as the *anal canal* (U). Three transverse folds project into the lumen of the rectum: *superior* (V_1), *middle* (V_2), and *inferior* (V_3) *rectal folds*.

ANAL CANAL

The anal canal, about 3 cm in length, features a large plexus of *hemorrhoidal veins* (W), as well as *internal* (X) and *external* (Y) *sphincter muscles*. Just prior to opening *anal columns* (Z), richly endowed with venous plexuses, are found. The inferior opening of the canal is the *anus* (ZZ).

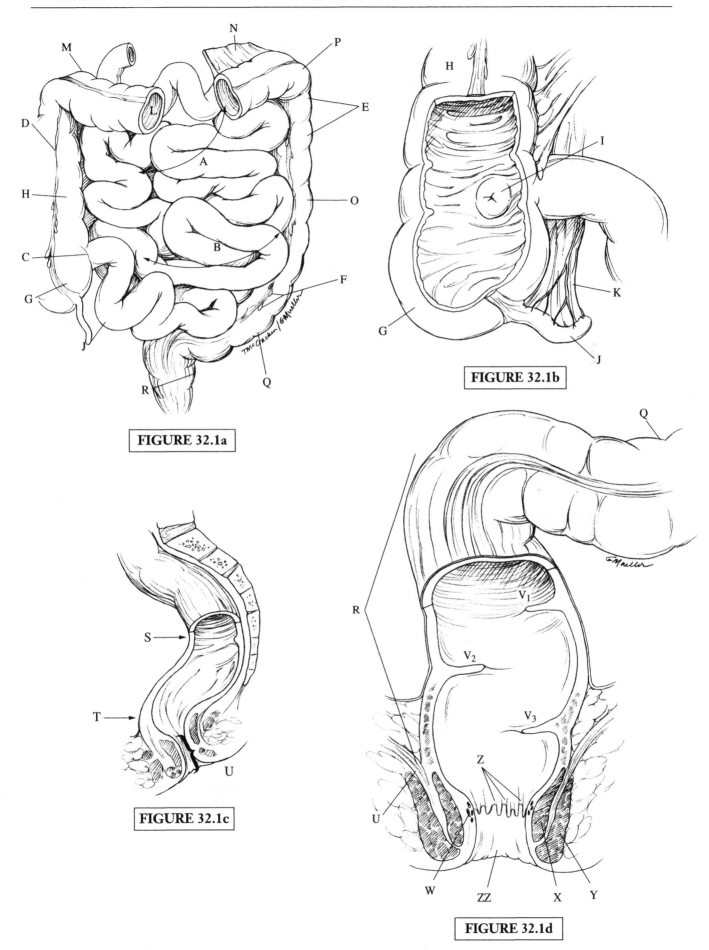

FIGURE 32.1a

FIGURE 32.1b

FIGURE 32.1c

FIGURE 32.1d

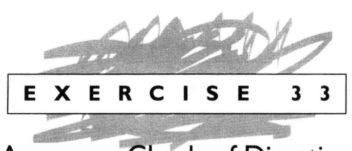

Accessory Glands of Digestion

ACCESSORY GLANDS

The *head of the pancreas* (A) (FIGURE 33.1a) is nestled in the curvature of the duodenum while the *body* (B) and *tail* (C) point to the left and the *spleen* (D). The superior mesenteric artery and vein appear from deep to this gland and pass anterior to the horizontal portion. Digestive enzymes secreted by the pancreas enter the duodenum via the greater and accessory (if present) pancreatic ducts.

The *liver* (E) is located superior to the first portion of the duodenum. It presents visceral and diaphragmatic surfaces and two main lobes (FIGURE 33.1b and 33.1c): a larger *right* (F) (color bar: red) and a smaller l*eft* (G) (color bar: orange). *Right* (H) and *left* (I) *hepatic ducts* leave their respective lobes to unite as the *common hepatic duct* (J) (color yellow). Two other lobes of note: the *quadrate* (F_1) and the *caudate* (F_2) are subdivisions of the right lobe. These are separated by the *porta hepatis* (K) through which the *portal vein* (L), *hepatic artery* (M), and hepatic ducts pass.

The diaphragmatic and visceral surfaces are associated with two blind peritoneal pouches (FIGURE 33.1d). The *subphrenic recess* (N) is found between the deep surface of the diaphragm and the superior surface of the liver. This pouch ends at the *coronary ligament* (O) (color sky blue), a reflection of the peritoneum from the deep surface of the diaphragm over the superior and anterior surfaces of the

liver. Between the right kidney and the liver is another peritoneal pouch: *the hepatorenal recess* (P). Peritoneum passes from the deep surface of the liver onto the anterior surface of the kidney. At the superior end of this pouch is the *hepatorenal ligament* (Q) (color violet). The area of the liver between these two "ligaments" is devoid of peritoneum and is known as the *bare area* (R) (color brown).

The *gall bladder* (S) is tucked neatly beneath the inferior surface of the liver, between the right and quadrate lobes. The blind end is the *fundus* (T_1), with a *body* (T_2), and *neck* (T_3) tapering to the *cystic duct* (U) (color blue). This duct is a short (2-4 cm) channel that meets the common hepatic duct to form the *common bile duct* (V) (color green), which usually unites with the pancreatic duct for a joint opening into the descending portion of the duodenum (see page 176).

The *spleen* (D) is a bit of a stretch as an accessory digestive gland but we'll give it a go! The spleen is appended to the greater curvature of the stomach via the *gastrolienal ligament* (X). It is also anchored to the left kidney by the *lienorenal ligament* (Y). The spleen functions in the destruction and removal of old red blood cells, a process setting free a breakdown product called bilirubin. This is delivered to the liver in the splenic vein via the hepatic portal system. The liver uses bilirubin in the production of bile!

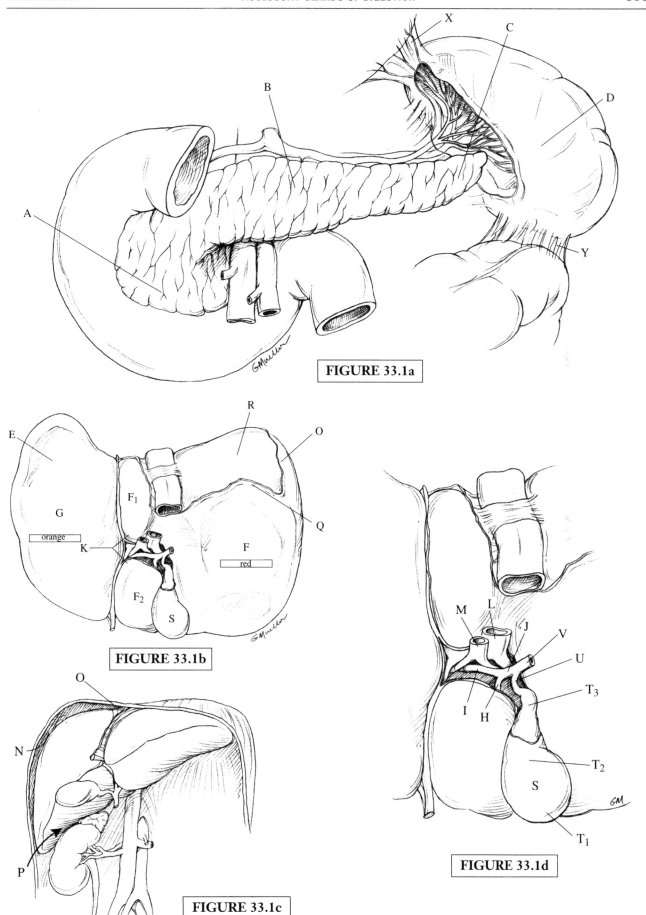

FIGURE 33.1a

FIGURE 33.1b

FIGURE 33.1c

FIGURE 33.1d

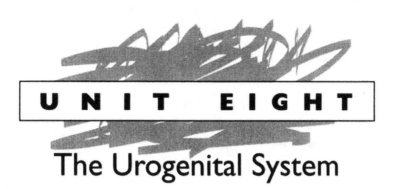

UNIT EIGHT

The Urogenital System

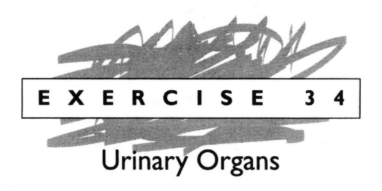

EXERCISE 34

Urinary Organs

KIDNEYS

The paired *kidneys* (A) (FIGURE 34.1a) are found retroperitoneally on the posterolateral abdominal wall; obscured by fat and fascia. The posterior surface of the kidneys is flattened while the anterior surface is somewhat convex. Each kidney has a *medial border* (B) with a concavity at the *hilus* (C); the point of entry and exit of renal vessels and the ureter. The convex *lateral border* (D) is unremarkable.

A hemisected kidney (FIGURE 34.1b and 34.1c) shows a number of important features. The *renal cortex* (E) is most external and consists of *glomeruli* (F) and *convoluted renal tubules* (G). The cortex extends into the *renal pelvis* (H) as *renal columns* (I). The *renal medulla* (J) is deep to the cortex and consists of a number of *renal pyramids* (K). The bases of these pyramids are at the junction of the cortical and medullary portions. The medial tips of the pyramids form *renal papillae* (L) which empty into 6-16 cup-shaped *minor renal calyces* (M) (color yellow). The minor calyces combine to form two or three *major calyces* (N) (color orange) in each kidney. These major calyces unite to form the renal pelvis (color red-orange) leading to the ureter.

The functional core of the urinary system is the *nephron* (O). The production of urine begins in the glomeruli. Between this point and the renal papillae a variety of active and passive transport systems function to preserve water and necessary chemical ions, while packaging ammonia wastes, drug metabolites, and other metabolic by-products for elimination.

URETERS

Passage of urine from the renal pelvis to the bladder is via paired *ureters* (P): muscular tubes approximately 25 cm long (FIGURE 34.1a) (color green). Each ureter has a very narrow lumen and a thick smooth muscled wall for movement of urine via peristaltic waves of contraction. In its passage to the bladder each ureter is described in abdominal and pelvic portions (each about one-half the total length). This entire descent is retroperitoneal.

The *abdominal portion of each ureter* (color red) is found along the anterior surface of the psoas major muscle. The *pelvic portion* (color yellow-green) begins as each ureter passes anterior to the external iliac artery, just distal to the bifurcation of the common iliac artery. Each passes posterior to the gonadal vessels to enter the posterosuperior angle of the urinary bladder.

❓ FOR REVIEW AND THOUGHT

Renal calculi (kidney stones) are an all too frequent feature of the human existence. Such calculi, composed of mineral salts (calcium oxalate, calcium phosphate, etc.) develop in the renal pelvis and may make their way down the ureter. Such movement is associated with excruciating pain know as ureteric colic caused by distention of the ureteric walls as the stone is moved via peristaltic waves. This pain may be referred to the inguinal region, the scrotum, or the labia.

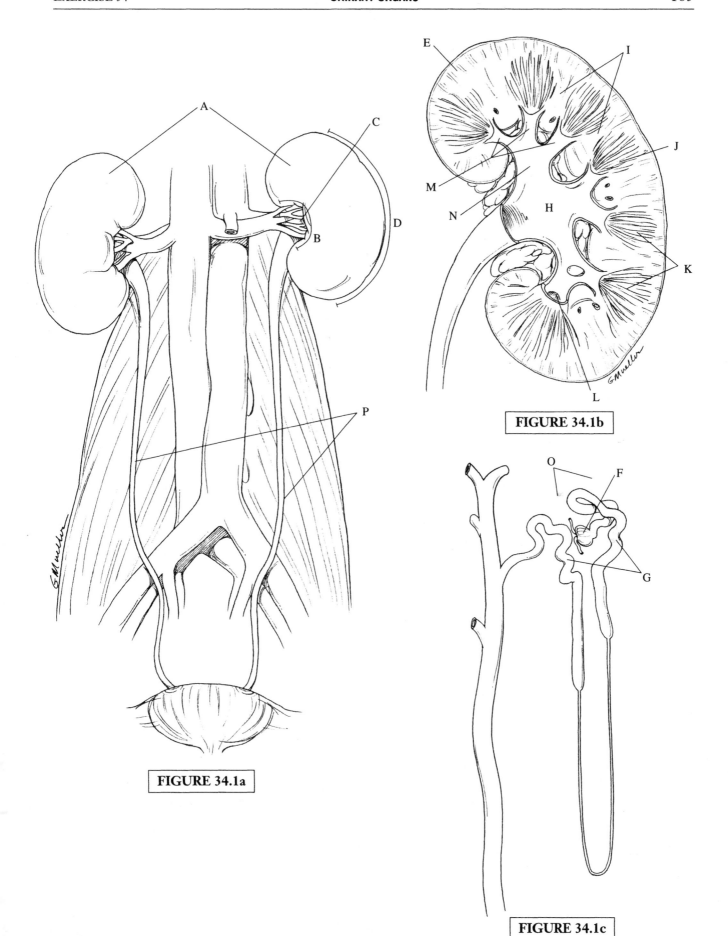

FIGURE 34.1a

FIGURE 34.1b

FIGURE 34.1c

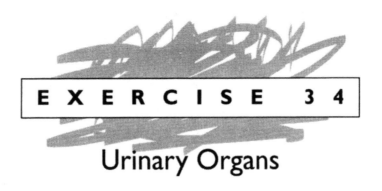

URINARY BLADDER

Posterior to the pubic bones the muscularly walled sac known as the *urinary bladder* (A) is found. The specifics of shape, size, and position of the bladder (FIGURES 34.2a and 34.2b) varies with age and the amount of urine contained. The superior surface of the bladder is covered by *parietal peritoneum* (B).

When empty the bladder is often described as having superior, posterior, and two inferolateral surfaces. The anterior point of the superior surface is the *apex* (C) and the posterior surface is the *base*, or *fundus* (D). The base and the inferolateral walls converge at the *neck* (E).

The interior of the bladder shows a *trigone* (F) between the terminal *openings of the ureters* (G) and the *internal urethral orifice* (H) (shade the trigone in yellow). This area appears smooth due to the tight attachment of the mucous membrane to the muscular wall of the bladder; in contrast to the remainder of the internal surface. Within the trigone find a slight median elevation: the *uvula of the bladder* (I).

The neck of the urinary bladder is supported inferiorly by a sling-like smooth muscle layer (FIGURE 34.2c). Three muscles comprise this structure. The *pubovesical* (J) (color green) passes from the deep surface of the pubic symphysis to surround the neck of the bladder. The *rectovesical* (K) (color sky blue) from the longitudinal musculature of the rectum to the lateral portion of the fundus of the bladder and the *rectourethral* (L) (color blue), from the longitudinal musculature of the rectum to the male urethra.

URETHRA

The urethra is the final common pathway for the voiding of urine in both sexes and ejaculation of semen in the male. The male urethra is characteristically about 15-20 cm in length. The internal urethral orifice is found at the anterior tip of the trigone of the bladder (see above). It is typically described in three parts.

The *prostatic portion* (color yellow), about 3 cm in length, passes through the prostate gland and is characterized by a median *urethral crest* (M) with grooves on each side: the *prostatic sinuses* (N). The ducts of the prostate gland empty into these sinuses or along the sides of the crest. The central portion of the crest shows a swelling, or eminence, the *seminal colliculus* (O). The tiny openings of the ejaculatory ducts are found on each side of the colliculus. The colliculus also shows a small opening leading posteriorly to a blind sac: the *prostatic utricle* (P). The utricle (L., a small sac) is a vestigial remnant of the embryonic uterovaginal canal and is homologous to the uterus and vagina in the female.

The urethra continues as the very short (1 cm) *membranous portion* (color orange). It passes from the apex of the prostate gland to pierce the sphincter urethrae muscle and the perineal membrane. The *bulbourethral glands* (Q) (color blue) are arranged on each side of this portion of the urethra.

The third, and longest (about 15 cm), is the *spongy portion* (R) (color red-orange). It begins at the point the urethra enters the corpus spongiosum of the penis and continues to the *external urethral orifice* (S_1). The ducts of the *bulbourethral glands* (Q_1) drain into the wall of the most proximal portion of this part of the spongy urethra. Because most of the length of this portion is contained within the structure of the penis it is often called the *penile urethra*.

The *female urethra* (FIGURE 34.2d) is quite short (2 to 6 cm), equating to the prostatic and membranous portions of the male. Its course from the bladder is anteroinferior and it opens via the *external urethral orifice* (S_2) between the labia minora, anterior to the vaginal orifice and posterior to the clitoris.

❓ FOR REVIEW AND THOUGHT

Trace a drop of urine from a minor calyx of the kidney to voiding.

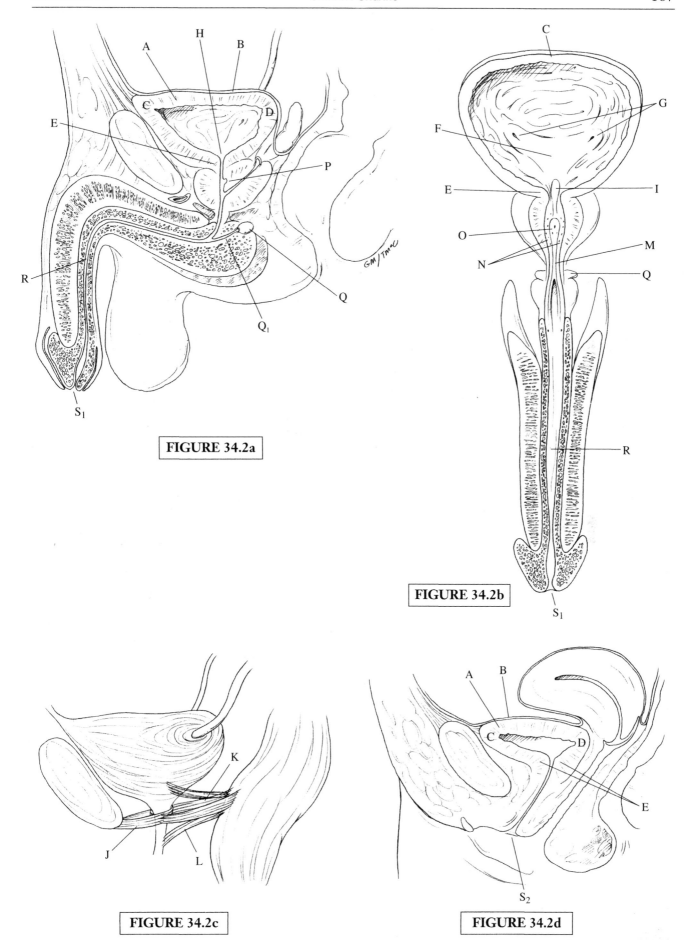

FIGURE 34.2a

FIGURE 34.2b

FIGURE 34.2c

FIGURE 34.2d

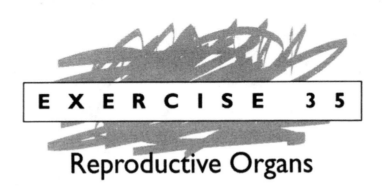

EXERCISE 35

Reproductive Organs

MALE

The male reproductive organs (testes and associated ducts) develop retroperitoneally near the kidneys, in the superolateral abdominal wall, in an area called the urogenital ridge. During the last trimester of embryonic development these structures descend to their adult site in the *scrotum* (A) (FIGURE 35.1a). In this descent the testes drag the vas deferens, testicular artery and vein, nerve supply, and lymphatics with them. These structures, together with the layers of the abdominal wall pierced during passage, in order to escape the warm environs of the abdomen, are known as the *spermatic cord* (B) (FIGURES 35.1a-c). In the female the *round ligament of the uterus* (C) takes this path (FIGURE 35.1c).

The components of the spermatic cord are layered upon one-another in a dictated sequence. The cord begins at the *deep inguinal ring* (D), a defect in the transversalis fascia produced by the protrusion of the *processus vaginalis* (E), to initiate what is to become the *inguinal canal* (F). From deep to superficial the layerings of the spermatic cord are:

internal spermatic fascia (B₁), derived from transversalis fascia (color green)
cremasteric fascia (B₂), derived from the internal oblique muscle and its fascia (color sky blue)
external spermatic fascia (B₃), from the aponeurosis of the external oblique muscle (color blue)

The *cremaster muscle* (G) is derived from scattered fibers of the internal oblique muscle. The fibers of the cremaster, not under voluntary control, reflexly draw the testis superiorly in the scrotum; back toward the warmth of the abdomen from which it fled during descent. Any male who has swum in cold water can attest to this cremasteric reflex!

TESTES

The *testes* (H) (FIGURE 35.1d) are oval-shaped glandular organs suspended in the scrotum by the spermatic cords. They function in both the production of spermatozoa and the male sex hormone testosterone. The external surface of the testis is the *tunica albuginea* (I) (color violet) with septa extending into the depth of the organ to create lobules of *seminiferous tubules* (J). Within these tubules spermatozoa are formed. At the tip of each lobule the seminiferous tubules converge to form *straight tubules* (K) which, in turn, join to form the *rete testis* (L). Fifteen to twenty *efferent ductules* (M) connect the rete testis to the head of the epididymis. *Appendices testis* (N) may be present on the exterior surface of the testis.

The *epididymis* (O) (color light brown) is perched upon the superior and posterolateral surface of the testis. Described portions of this structure include the *head* (O₁), *body* (O₂), and *tail* (O₃). The body of the epididymis is greatly convoluted and serves as a storage site for sperm during their final maturation. The tail of the epididymis is continuous with the *ductus (vas) deferens* (P) (color yellow), which transports sperm to the *ejaculatory duct* (Q) (color red-orange) for passage into the urethra.

Two interesting items are associated with the head of the epididymis. The *sinus of the epididymis* (R) is a pouch-like recess between the head and the surface of the testis. One, or more, *appendices of the epididymis* (S) may also be found.

🌙 JUST FOR FUN!

What is the difference between the tail of the epididymis and the ejaculatory duct? There is a vas deferens between them!

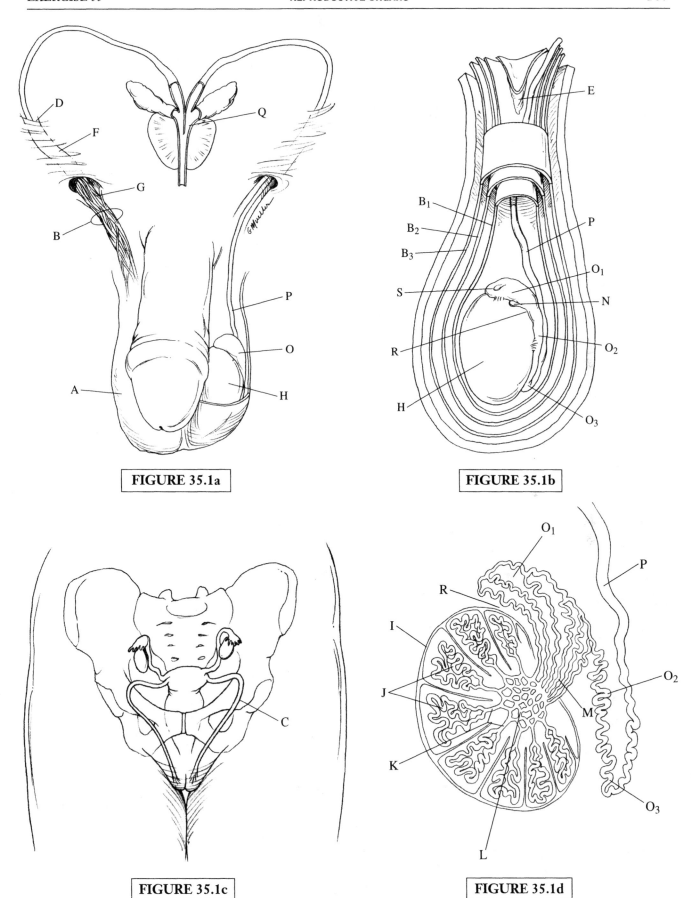

FIGURE 35.1a

FIGURE 35.1b

FIGURE 35.1c

FIGURE 35.1d

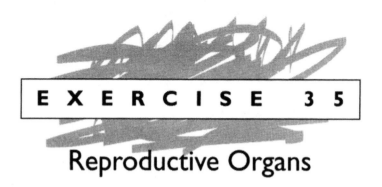

EXERCISE 35

Reproductive Organs

MALE

Vas Deferens

Each *ductus (vas) deferens* (A) (color yellow) (FIGURES 35.2a and 35.2b) ascends within the spermatic cord through the inguinal canal and into the pelvis to empty into the prostatic portion of the urethra. In this course it is quite superficial and palpable in the scrotum (explaining the relative ease of vasectomy).

After entering the abdominal cavity each vas deferens passes superior to the ureter and posterior to the bladder to converge on the base of the bladder (FIGURE 35.2b). At this point each swells slightly as the *ampulla* (A_1). The *seminal vesicle* (more correctly, the *seminal gland)* (B) (color orange) joins here via an *excretory duct* (B_1) (color red) to form a common *ejaculatory duct* (C) (color red-orange) emptying into the prostatic portion of the urethra.

Associated Glands

The seminal gland is one of three accessory glands involved in producing an ejaculate capable of surviving the hostile environment of the female reproductive tract. It produces a thick secretion thought to be involved in activation of spermatozoa.

The *prostate gland* (D) (color green) is a chestnut-sized and shaped organ composed of multiple tubuloalveolar glands. It surrounds the base of the penis and produces a secretion containing alkaline enzymes to counteract the acidity of the vagina and to increase sperm motility. Its secretion enters the urethra via the prostatic sinuses. Paired *bulbourethral (Cowper's) glands* (E) (color yellow-green) are found in the urogenital diaphragm and secrete a mucus product via short ducts emptying into the spongy portion of the urethra.

Penis

The male sexual organ is the *penis* (F) (FIGURE 35.2c). It is composed of three separate erectile bodies. Paired *corpora cavernosa penis* (F_1) (color blue) are shown with a single *corpus spongiosum penis* (F_2) (color violet) between and ventral.

The corpora cavernosa are attached to the medial surfaces of the pubic arch via *crura* (legs) (F_3) allowing support for the more inferior spongiosum portion. The *root of the penis* (F_4) is the attached portion consisting of the two crura, the *bulb of the penis* (F_5), and associated muscles. The bulb is the origin of the spongiosum portion from the perineal space and membrane. The bulb is pierced by the beginning of the urethra as it exits the bladder. The penile portion of the urethra is in the spongiosum portion of the penis. The three corpora form the *body* (F_6) of the penis. The distal end of the corpus spongiosum penis is the *glans penis* (F_7) (color light brown).

A *prepuce* (foreskin) (F_8) covers the glans penis to some extent. The *frenulum of the prepuce* (F_9) is found on the undersurface of the glans. The glans also shows the *external urethral orifice* (F_{10}).

❓ FOR REVIEW AND THOUGHT

Circumcision

Part or all the prepuce is removed routinely on nearly all newborn males in North America. To Jews circumcision is much more than a surgical procedure. It is an extremely important religious rite that must be done on the 8th day and in accordance with ancient traditions and procedures.

Erection

Erection of the penis is a parasympathetically controlled event brought about by the engorgement of the corpora cavernosa with blood. This process decreases peripheral venous return resulting in enlargement and rigidity of the cavernosa. This response is not as pronounced in the spongiosum allowing the urethra to remain patent for the ejaculation of semen at orgasm.

You should be able to trace spermatozoa from their site of production through the genital structures to their site of ejaculation, naming all accessory glands along their course.

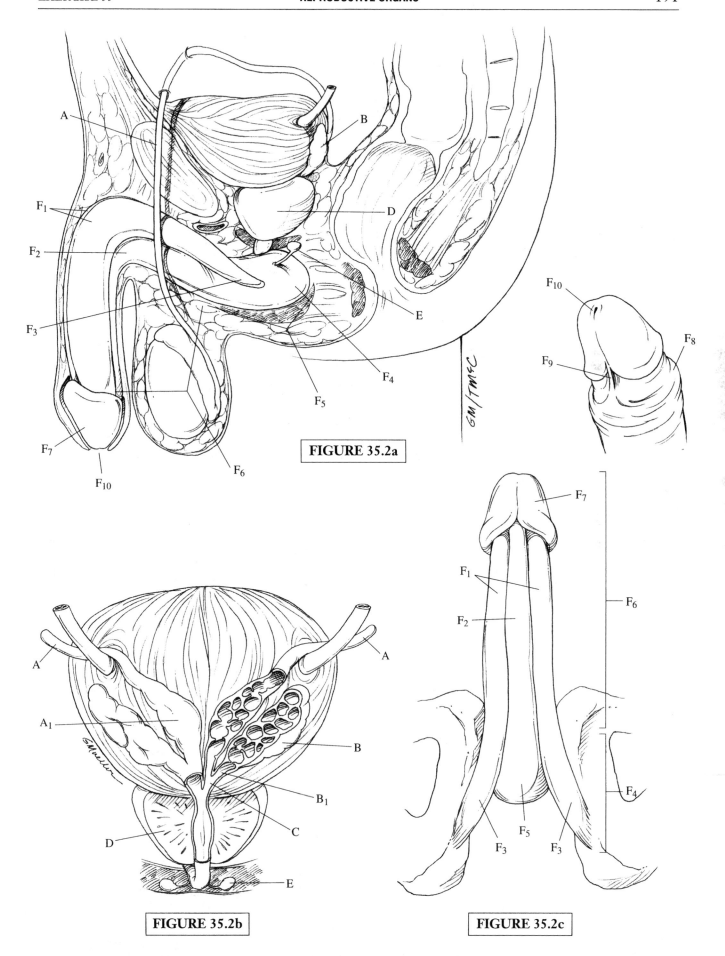

FIGURE 35.2a

FIGURE 35.2b

FIGURE 35.2c

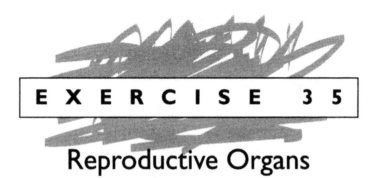

EXERCISE 35

Reproductive Organs

FEMALE

Uterus

The *uterus* (A) (FIGURE 35.3a and 35.3b) is described in three portions: *body* (A$_1$), *fundus* (A$_2$), and *cervix* (A$_3$), and with *right and left margins* (A$_4$): in actuality the lateral borders. The body has a *cavity* (A$_5$) lined with mucus membrane. The fundus is the dome of the uterus superior to the entrance of the uterine tubes. The inferior portion is the *cervix*. It is this portion that communicates with the *vagina* (B) via the *orifice of the uterus* (C). Note how this orifice 'dips' into the superior end of the vagina forming blind pouches both anteriorly and posteriorly, with the latter being much more prominent. These are the *anterior fornix* (D) (outline in yellow) and *posterior fornix* (E) (outline in orange). Anterior to the vagina is the *urethra* (F) and posterior is the *rectum* (G).

Note the position of the uterus! The cervix is bent anteriorly in relationship to the vaginal fornices. This is described as *anteflexion*! The uterus as a whole is also usually bent forward over the bladder. This is described as *anteversion*. The anteflexed and anteverted position of the uterus is the most common.

Our discussion of uterine position gains importance when we consider the peritoneal reflections over the bladder, uterus, and anterior surface of the rectum. Note that the anteverted/anteflexed position produces peritoneal pouches between the uterus and bladder (*vesicouterine* [H], outline in red-orange), and between the uterus and rectum (*rectouterine* [I], outline in red). Though the uterus is retroperitoneal it is supported laterally by a sheet of peritoneum known as the *broad ligament* (J) (color yellow-green). The uterine tubes and ovary are found in the posterior edge of this ligament. The anterior edge of the broad ligament presents the round ligament of the uterus.

The *uterine (Fallopian) tubes* (K) (color green) extend laterally from the body of the uterus. Each is described in three portions: *uterine* (K$_1$), located in the uterine wall; *isthmus* (K$_2$), the narrowest portion; and the largest portion, the *ampullar* (K$_3$), comprises the lateral half of the length of the tube. At its end the tube enlarges greatly as the *ampulla* (K$_4$) and shows an opening, the *ostium* (K$_5$), surrounded by a multitude of finger-like appendages, the *fimbriae* (K$_6$).

Ovaries

Like the testes the ovaries develop retroperitoneally in the superolateral wall of the abdomen and descend to the pelvis in the last trimester dragging vessels and nerves. They do not, however, leave the abdomen: as did the testes. This process is so similar that the female retains an 'equivalent' to the spermatic cord: the *round ligament of the uterus* (L) (color sky blue). It is found in the anterior portion of the broad ligament. Analogous to the spermatic cord in the male this ligament dissolves into fibrous connective tissue in the labia. The *ligament of the ovary* (M) (color violet) is found in the posterior portion of the broad ligament.

External Female Genitalia

Two pairs of lips obscure the entrance to the vagina (FIGURE 35.3c). The *labii majora* (N) (color light brown) are equivalent to the scrotum in the male. The *labii minora* (O) enclose the opening into the vagina; an area known as the *vestibule* (P). Follow the rim of the labii minora anteriorly to find the *glans clitoris* (Q) (color brown), enclosed within a division of the labii minora. The anterior portion of this division forms the *frenulum* (R) and the posterior the *prepuce* (S).

The clitoris consists of two corpora cavernosa attached to the pubic arch via crura, like the penis, and is erectile during sexual stimulation. Paired *greater vestibular glands (Bartholin's glands)* (T) (color yellow), homologous to the bulbourethral gland of the male, secrete a mucus fluid into the labial area.

Vagina

This flattened tube leading to the uterus is approximately 10 cm in length and presents *anterior* (U) and *posterior* (V) walls. The protrusion of the cervix into the superior end of the vagina, forming fornices, has already been discussed. The vagina lies between the urinary bladder anteriorly and the rectum posteriorly. In the virgin the entrance to the vagina is partially or wholly occluded by a membranous fold: *the hymen*.

❓ FOR REVIEW AND THOUGHT

What is the most common position of the uterus? What is meant by a tubal pregnancy? Where are the fornices of the vagina and what is their significance?

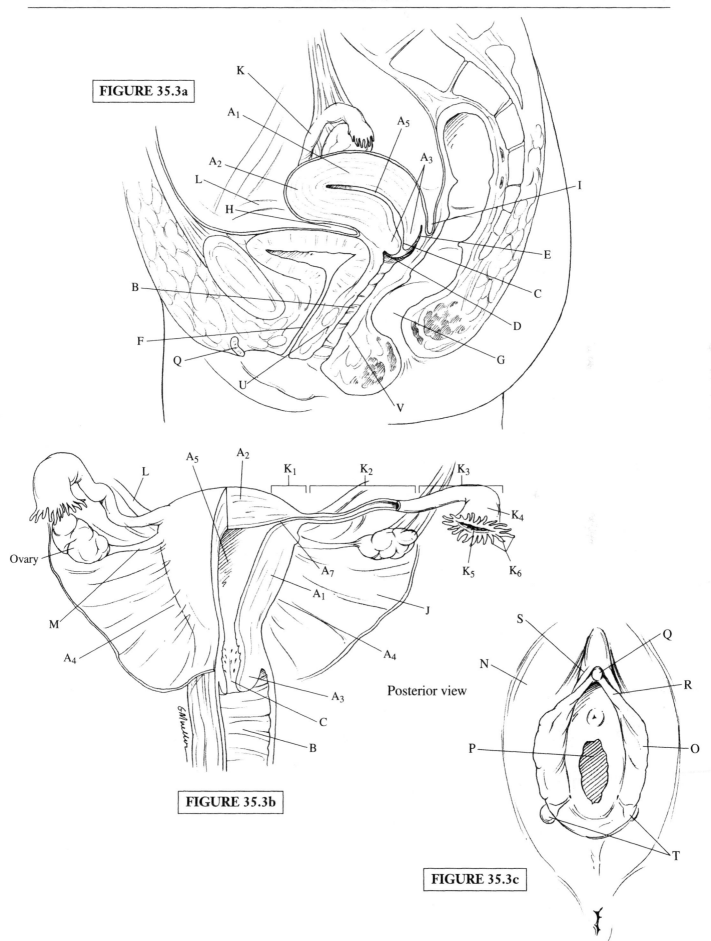

FIGURE 35.3a

FIGURE 35.3b

Posterior view

FIGURE 35.3c

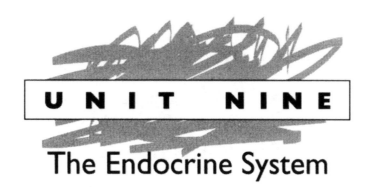

UNIT NINE

The Endocrine System

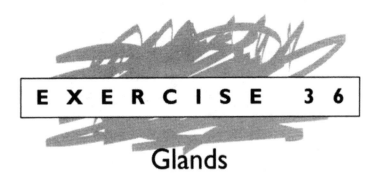

EXERCISE 36

Glands

Endocrine glands are found in the head, neck, and trunk. While differing in size, location, function, and targets they all have two things in common: they are ductless and they dispatch their product (hormones) directly into the bloodstream.

PITUITARY GLAND

The *pituitary gland* (A) (FIGURE 36.1) hangs suspended from the hypothalamus. It is the 'rider' in the sella turcica (see page 34) and the most influential of all the endocrine glands. It is structurally and functionally divided into a larger *anterior* (A_1) (shade in yellow) and smaller *posterior lobe* (A_2) (shade in orange). Hormone production by the anterior lobe (often referred to as the adenohypophysis or glandular lobe) is influenced by hypothalamic releasing factors. The list of anterior lobe hormones is indeed significant!

Anterior Lobe

Growth hormone (GH) – exerts a direct effect on protein, lipid, and carbohydrate metabolism and controls the rate of visceral and skeletal growth.
Adrenocorticotropic hormone (ACTH) – exerts a stimulatory effect on the release of glucocorticoid hormones from the adrenal glands.
Thyroid-stimulating hormone (TSH) – also called thyrotropin; stimulates production and release of thyroid hormone by the thyroid gland.
Follicle-stimulating hormone (FSH) – stimulates maturation of ova and the release of estrogen by the ovaries; stimulates sperm production in the testes.
Luteinizing hormone – acts with FSH to cause ovulation and the production of progesterone in the ovary; also stimulates testosterone production in the testes.
Prolactin – stimulates and sustains lactation postpartum.

Posterior Lobe

This portion of the pituitary gland is often referred to as the neurohypophysis or neural lobe! Its hormones are fewer in number and quite specific in action.

Oxytocin – stimulates uterine contraction during child-birth; stimulates the mammary glands to release milk.
Antidiuretic hormone (vasopressin) – promotes retention of water in the kidneys; acts to increase blood pressure via vasoconstriction of arterioles.

Thyroid Gland

This gland (B) (FIGURE 36.2a) is positioned in a U shape just inferior to the thyroid cartilage. It shows ascending *right and left lobes* (B_1) connected by a narrow isthmus (B_2). Occasionally a vestigial *pyramidal lobe* (B_3) is found ascending toward the hyoid bone. The gland secretes, stores, and releases three hormones (color this gland green).

Thyroxin and Triiodothyronine – together these are referred to as 'thyroid hormone'; they function in regulating metabolic rate; hormone release is controlled by the anterior lobe of the pituitary via TSH.
Calcitonin – functions to decrease blood calcium levels; works in concert with parathyroid hormone.

Parathyroid Glands

Four tiny glands (C) (FIGURE 36.2b) are found embedded in the posterior surface of the thyroid gland. They are often described as *superior* (C_1) and *inferior* (C_2) pairs (shade in sky blue). Parathyroid hormone acts to increase blood calcium levels.

Thymus

The *thymus* (D) (FIGURE 36.3) is a prominent constituent of the mediastinum in youth. It is usually found directly posterior to the manubrium. With the onset of puberty this gland begins to atrophy and by adulthood is virtually impossible to find. During its youthful existence it functions in the development and maturation of cell-mediated immunologic activities.

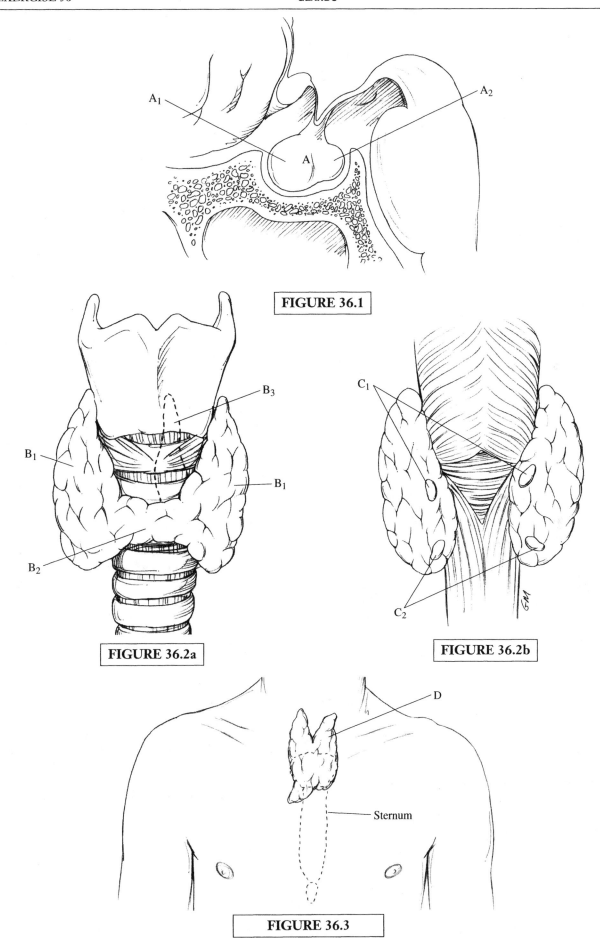

FIGURE 36.1

FIGURE 36.2a

FIGURE 36.2b

Sternum

FIGURE 36.3

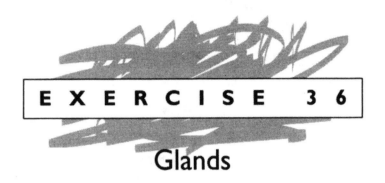

EXERCISE 36
Glands

ADRENAL GLANDS

The *adrenal glands* (A) (FIGURE 36.4a and 36.4b) are found perched upon the superior poles of the kidneys. These glands are composed of superficial *cortical* (A$_1$) and deep *medullary* (A$_2$) portions. In point of fact these two portions function as separate glands.

The cortical portion (color yellow) produces steroid hormones under the control of the pituitary gland: via ACTH.

Glucocorticoids – the most significant being cortisol, which aids the body in adapting to changing or threatening conditions

Mineralocorticoids – aldosterone, for example; controls the level of sodium and potassium in the blood; and limits the loss of sodium in the urine

Gonadocorticoids – estrogens and androgens

The medullary portion (color orange) produces catecholamine hormones (epinephrine and norepinephrine) in response to activation of the autonomic nervous system. These hormones produce the fight-or-flight response and are short-lived in action.

PANCREAS

This organ (B) (FIGURE 36.5a) is unique in having both exocrine and endocrine functions. Description of the exocrine function in digestion was covered in Exercise 32. Approximately 99% of the composition of this gland is devoted to its exocrine role, a fact that makes it endocrine role even more remarkable. Scattered within the substance of the gland are small collections of specialized cells for the synthesis and secretion of insulin or glucagon. These gatherings of like-cells are the *Islets of Langerhans* (B$_1$) (shade in violet) (FIGURE 36.5b).

Insulin – produced by beta cells in the Islets in response to elevated blood glucose; functions to limit blood glucose by stimulating glucose uptake into skeletal muscle, liver, and adipose tissue.

Glucagon – produced by alpha cells in the Islets in response to decreased levels of blood glucose; functions to increase blood glucose by stimulating the conversion of glycogen to glucose in the liver

OVARIES

The *ovaries* (C) (FIGURE 36.6) secrete estrogen and progesterone for the purpose of maintaining the reproductive system and for preparing this sytem, and the body, for pregnancy. Both of these hormones are under the control of FSH and LH.

Estrogen – produces secondary sex characteristics (growth of breasts, fat deposition, widening of the hips, etc.); functions with growth hormone during puberty to promote general growth.

Progesterone – prepares the endometrium of the uterus for the receipt of a fertilized ovum.

TESTES

In addition to their role in producing spermatozoa the *testes* (D) (FIGURE 36.7a) (shade in blue) produce a powerful steroid hormone. Testosterone is secreted by specialized *Leydig Cells* (D$_1$) (FIGURE 36.7b) surrounding the seminiferous tubules.

Testosterone – produces male secondary sex characteristics and maintains them in adulthood; a significant ally of growth hormone during puberty; maintains the libido (sex drive).

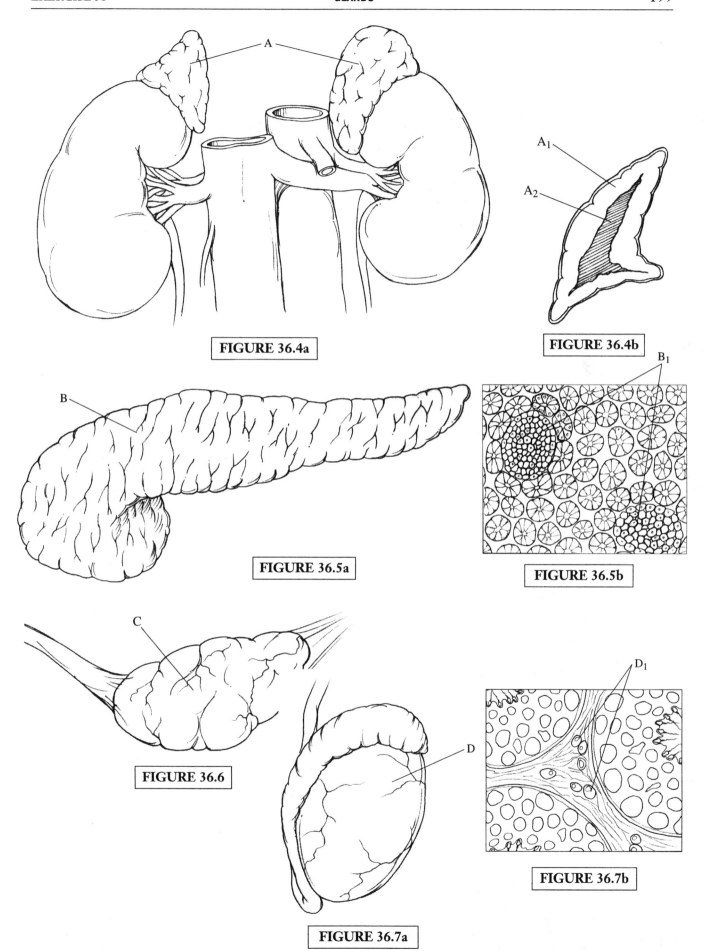

FIGURE 36.4a

FIGURE 36.4b

FIGURE 36.5a

FIGURE 36.5b

FIGURE 36.6

FIGURE 36.7a

FIGURE 36.7b

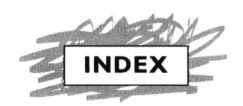

INDEX